KNOW YOUR ENEMY:
THE CANCER

KNOW YOUR ENEMY:
THE CANCER

Natural Therapies, Healing Techniques and Testimonies

EVA L. GREEN, BSc, CYTOLOGIST

Library of Congress Control Number: 2015910508
ISBN: Hardcover   978-1-5035-0688-6
                   Softcover   978-1-5035-0689-3
                   eBook   978-1-5035-0690-9

This book is a collection of documents and information regarding the nonconventional therapies for cancer made by numerous scientists all over the world and has no intention to convince you to stop or change your treatment. It also contains testimonies made by doctors and usual people like you and me on natural therapies which managed to save their lives, and it is your choice to believe them or not.

It is up to you to consider these pieces of information, to do your own research in this regard, and to apply the knowledge gained to your benefit. And like always in life, you have a choice to make from various options lined up in front of you, and you need to decide based on your level of understanding and consciousness what is the best thing which will serve your interest.

Print information available on the last page.

Rev. date: 07/07/2015

I dedicate this book to my two sons, Theo and Eddy, the greatest treasure in my life, with gratitude for sharing this hard journey with me and contributing to my healing and spiritual evolution; to Doctor Coralia Jigau, who sacrificed her time and energy to help me and other ill people with a dedication rarely seen; and to all the people crossing my life's path who, in one way or the other, have influenced my journey.

FOREWORD

'The wound is the place where the Light enters you' (Rumi).

We all go through challenges, whether personal or universal. One of the biggest challenges that has found its way into everyone's life is the all-feared cancer. If you or a loved one has been through such a challenge, you will be all too acquainted with the cold fear and deep wounds it has the potential to create on all levels of the being—*potential* being the key word.

However, I've heard many people discuss in the aftermath of such an illness that, in fact, it was sent in one's life as a miracle, as a way of opening the doors to an infinite world of learning, growing, and inspiring. How can we as human beings, without what seems to be potent struggle, grow and learn to deeply appreciate *life* and all things in it? Human nature is such that until we experience pain, we know not how to really love and see the beauty.

So this wonderful book talks of the journey of a dear friend who, after being diagnosed with breast cancer in 2012, decided to take the reins on this wild horse and make profound changes in her life physically, emotionally, and spiritually.

This book is an amalgamation of all the learning throughout this battle.

Thank you for sharing your story, Eva.

Lilly Leah Stesin

CONTENTS

No attempt should be made to cure the body without (curing) the soul.

Plato

In order to facilitate healing, it is important to explore the relationship between body, mind and spirit.

Dr David R. Hawkins

All our dreams can come true, if we have the courage to pursue them.

Walt Disney

INTRODUCTION

The day when I was diagnosed with cancer in 2012 was the 'switch' which changed my life in all its aspects.

In that moment, you will feel lost (as the society teaches us to feel) and like nothing on earth can help you, as all your dreams come to an end once they put the cancer label on you. You are condemned to death, and nothing else matters! The memories of the past have no value anymore and the future plans are all erased in that second. You have been a spark which now will disappear.

This is the first feeling when you get the news, and it is very important to pass it and to pay attention to the second thought, which says, 'What if there is a way out of this?' Sometimes, the second feeling comes much later, but it is the key to open the door for your healing.

As soon as you get rid of the idea of dying, your body will start to heal. The part of you which refuses to die starts screaming for help, starts searching, and the universe will send all the information and help your way; that's why you are reading this book.

Usually, the first person to ask help from is the doctor, which I did, and I was lucky that my GP, Dr Coralia Jigau in Melbourne, has a vast knowledge of the natural therapy. She helped me a lot in my journey, and I can say that she saved my life; but if you don't have a collaborative GP, search for a naturopath, or just follow the information in this book, in other books, or on the Internet. Check if they are accurate, and you can heal yourself.

Unfortunately, there are some obscure interests in the health system management in collaboration with the great pharmaceutical companies, which paradoxically don't wish you to become healthy because if you are sick, you are their source of income.

On the other hand, medical schools don't teach doctors to stay in touch with nature and use her healing power as the ancient healers did, but they teach them how to drug people with more and more chemicals in order to make profits for the pharmaceuticals companies—it is all a vicious circle.

It is hard to believe, but think that if there are people who kill others for $20, there are people who can do it for billions of dollars. It is not a paranoiac obsession or a conspiracy theory; it is the reality around us, and if you are looking closely, you will notice it.

If you are doing a quick research, you will find out that the treatment for cancer was discovered and used a long time ago but was restrained and hidden because it was too accessible and cheap with no profits for our money-craving brothers; so they made extracts of those natural remedies, put them in pills or injections, and made money from them, hiding that the origin of those products were actually in nature, free for everybody to use.

It is gladdening to see though how people are awakening and stop taking pills, which mask the effect of a disease but does not solve the cause of it, and returning to nature, which has all the resources we need to be healthy. There are more and more testimonials on the Internet and books about cancer cure, and I will present some of them in this book.

So in my despair to survive, I started searching for the *truth* about cancer because even though I had worked for twenty years in the medical field and screening cancers, I never was taught anything about the real cause or cure of cancer. The only treatments which I knew were chemotherapy, radiation, and operation.

There were on the Internet many natural treatments, but my science background didn't let me trust them until I understood their effect at the cellular level and read about the trials made on them.

I looked for a book to read about everything on the cause of cancer, alternative therapies, and some successful stories, but I didn't find one, and the information was scattered; it took almost one year to collect them, time in which the breast cancer had spread and metastasized in the bones.

That was the moment when I decided to help other people searching for the truth about cancer find all the information in one spot and understand why diet is important, how the substances we introduce in our body are transformed and work towards our healing, what is promoting cancer, and how we can kill cancer cells without damaging the good cells with chemotherapy. I wanted to clean the pathway in this jungle of information about the natural treatment for cancer.

All the information I found are collected in this book, and I hope that will save your time (the most precious asset in this fight) and will be useful for you like a good weapon in your battle with cancer or in helping others in their battle.

Yes, curing cancer, is a battle which requires discipline, commitment, and a very strong will to survive. The good news is that it is in your absolute power to live or die; it is your own choice. You choose to live . . . or die.

All our life, we have to choose between situations, people, and places.

Everything in life is a choice, and we live with the consequences of our choices; that is *free will*.

You decide what you want and how you wish to live your life, and the universe/God will say *yes* to your choice. Quantum mechanics scientifically explains this process (see chapter 4 of this book).

If you wish to be a prosperous winner, it's okay. If you wish to be a victim complaining all the time how unlucky and unfortunate you are, it's okay. It is up to you to choose how to live. You say/think it, and the universe will create it.

When you are diagnosed with cancer, it is the same. You choose to live or to die, and the universe/God will say yes to your choice. If you keep saying 'I have only six months to live' because the oncologist told you that (as he told me), you will program your body to live only six months, not more.

Become your own doctor and heal your cancer. You have multiple choices—the hard, unnatural, human-made suffering way of chemotherapy, radiation, and surgery or the natural, easy healing way offered by nature. You can choose!

It is up to you if you buy in and believe the society's perception that a person with cancer will die no matter what or if you open your eyes and search around for methods to fight cancer other than chemotherapy (which data shows is only 2 per cent successful) and look for real people who got out victorious from this fight. When you start searching for books, research documents, and Internet publications or videos, you will realize that there is a whole world out there very different from what you were taught. There are many cancer survivors, and you can be one of them.

The feeling of uselessness and hopelessness in front of death when it is knocking at your door is indescribable and only the people who have been there can understand that feeling.

At that moment, you realize that nothing, nothing at all, from the past matters, and all the things around you become meaningless and will vanish together with you, as the future doesn't exist any more.

This is the moment when you wake up from this long dream called life and start to live your reality. Only when you hit the wall in a life threatening event are you able to ask the magic question, Why?

Why me? Why has this disease or problem happened to me? What have I done wrong to my body, to my life, to my spirit that this anomaly was created?

You must consider yourself lucky to be able to ask this question and to start searching for answers.

Some people in that situation don't ask; they accept the diagnosis as a death sentence and lose their hope of living. They take drugs, undergo chemotherapy (which will damage more the weakened body), and eventually, they will die. Or they have to pass again and again that shocking moment until they wake up and ask why.

This question is the key to a magic door: the door to eternal life.

Now, because you have asked and started to search for answers (otherwise, you would not be reading this book and others which will follow), you have offered yourself a chance to live and to understand the meaning of life.

You will understand that (as it is described in the book *A Course in Miracles*) 'death is, a thought that takes on many forms, often unrecognised. It may appear as sadness, fear, anxiety, guilt, or doubt; as anger, faithlessness and lack of trust; concern for bodies, envy and all forms in which the wish to be as you are not, may come to tempt you'.

You will understand that we are marvellous creatures knitted from energy and matter by the marvellous Creator and our bodies have the power to regenerate and heal themselves if we keep them in harmony and balance with nature.

God created us in His image and similitude, so we must be perfect, and we are, but we have forgotten that.

Only now, when this threatening event has come to wake you up, will you start to ask: Where did I come from? Why do I have to die now? Will I have another life? Is this short life all that it is? How I can get another chance? How I can heal this disease? Why has this cancer formed in my body?

The answer to those questions exist; you can find them, and your search starts *now*!

CHAPTER 1

THE BODY

Our body is a perfect mechanism, a machinery ingeniously made in which all parts are interdependent and work in harmony through an energetic and chemical network to sustain life.

If a component of this complex 'machinery' is damaged, all others come to help and heal, taking minerals and nutrients from other sides and bringing them to the needing place to facilitate the healing. The human body is designed to heal itself. Every year, 98 per cent of the atoms in our body are exchanged for new atoms. You are constantly dying and being reborn and literally transforming at the atomic and molecular levels. Every three days, you have a new stomach lining; every month, you have new skin; every three months, you have a new skeleton; and every year, you have *almost an entirely new body* thanks to a perfectly working metabolic system. Keep this in mind and read it again and again in your fight with cancer. Knowing that your body has the power to regenerate and heal itself will empower you; you just need to learn how to help it by giving the necessary rebuilding materials/substances.

Everyone produces cancer cells in their body during a lifetime. Most people's immune systems have the resources available to take care of them. People with cancer have simply reached the stage that their immune system is so overworked and weakened that it has no resources left to take care of the cancer.

In order to cure cancer, we need to have knowledge about our 'enemy' and to know the cause of its development, its likes and dislikes, and we also need to know the connection between our actions, diet, behaviour, and our body's well-being.

The holistic approach of the body is the core to our healing success.

To understand how our body is functioning and to be confident that we can intervene, improve, modify its function, and heal ourselves, we need to learn a bit about our physiology.

I don't intend to write here a biology lesson. I just wish to make you understand how our body works so you will be confident to interfere, change, and help it to cure the cancer.

Let's have a journey through our body!

The physical body consists of three main parts:

1. the *cells*, which form tissues and organs
2. the *blood*
3. the *lymph*.

1. The Cells

Let's talk about the cells!

A cell is like a whole factory in which life is created and sustained in every single second. Thousands of chemical reactions are happening in every day in our body, transforming the ingested food in substances necessary for our existence.

It's said that there are approximately 100 trillion cells in a human body, and millions of them are being formed and dying every day.

Our bodies contain about 200 different types of cells, and each of them has inside almost 20 different types of organelles, which contribute to the cell function like little workers in a factory.

A human cell looks like this:

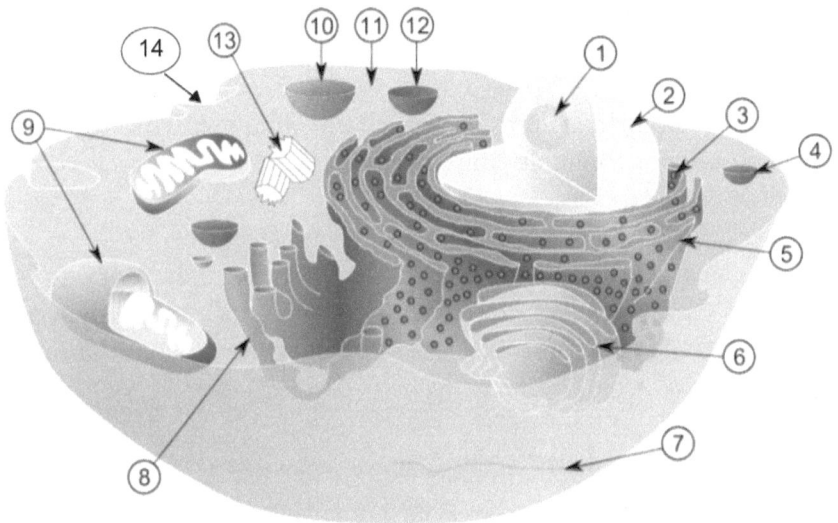

(http://commons.wikimedia.org/wiki/File:Biological_cell.svg)

1. nucleolus
2. nucleus
3. ribosome
4. vesicle
5. rough endoplasmic reticulum
6. Golgi apparatus
7. cytoskeleton
8. smooth endoplasmic reticulum
9. mitochondria
10. vacuole
11. cytoplasm
12. lysosome
13. centrioles
14. cell membrane.

Each cell has four major components: membrane, cytoplasm, nucleus, and cellular organelles.

At the exterior of the cell is the cell membrane, which protects the cell, forming a barrier between it and the environment. The membrane is made from proteins and lipids and lets the minerals and other substances get in and out of the cell. Cancer causes a decrease in the levels of integral membrane proteins and an increase in the levels of phospholipids. It might also lead to the reconstruction and functional rearrangement of the cell membrane, for example, the permeability, electric properties, fluidity, etc. Based on this observation, some natural therapies recommend the use of enzymes (pancreatic or gastric) to help penetrate the cell membrane and destroy the cancerous cell.

The cytoplasm is situated inside the cell membrane. It is a clear, thick, jelly material which contains the cytoskeleton and supports and protects all cell organelles.

The nucleus is the information centre of the cell. It contains the nucleolus (1, 2), controls cell activities, and contains the DNA, the hereditary material of the cell. Cells continually divide, contributing to the growth and repair of the body.

The organelles are situated in the cytoplasm and have distinct functions:

- nucleolus—situated in the nucleus, the site of ribosome synthesis
- ribosomes—create proteins
- vacuoles—store food, water, metabolic and toxic wastes
- Golgi apparatus—synthesizes, packages, and releases concentrated proteins or lipids
- rough endoplasmic reticulum—synthesizes enzymes and other proteins
- smooth endoplasmic reticulum—creates lipids or fat
- mitochondria—breaks down sugar (glucose) molecules to release energy, site of aerobic cellular respiration and energy storage
- liposome—small membrane bounded transport vesicles
- centrioles—paired structures near the nucleus which separate chromosome pairs during mitosis (cellular division and cellular reproduction)
- cytoskeleton—a system of microtubules which strengthens the cell, maintains the shape, and moves organelles within the cell
- lysosomes—contain hydrolytic enzymes for digestion.

All those organelles work together like the workers in a factory to maintain the chemical balance of the body. Each of them has a function and a to-do program.

Did you ever wonder how the body uses and transforms the food, the water, and the air to build muscles and bones? What happens when the cells ignore the patterns of building and create mutations? Why do those mutations occur?

Briefly, everything happens like this: In the metabolism process, through a series of chemical reactions, our body uses oxygen from the air to break down the nutrients which we take from the food in order to produce energy necessary to all the functions of the body. This energy is stored in the mitochondria, which is also called the energy keeper of the cell.

In the absence or restriction of oxygen, all those chemical reactions are slowed down or disturbed.

That's why you need a lot of oxygen to sustain the metabolism in the body. Also remember that the cancer cells do not like oxygen!

In our body, each type of cell has different jobs, and the cells with the same structure and function combine together to form tissue. The tissue with the same function form organs like lungs, liver, brain, etc. The organs specialized to do the same job form systems like the circulatory system, urinary system, reproductive system, etc. All the systems in our body are connected and work harmoniously to keep our body alive, and they perform certain duties.

- integumentary system
  o largest sensory organ
  o synthesizes vitamin D
  o protects deeper tissue
  o regulates fluid and blood loss.

- skeletal system
  o stores calcium
  o framework for the body

- o protects vital organs
- o produces red blood cells.

- muscular system
  - o generates heat
  - o creates movement
  - o maintains posture
  - o uses energy.

- immune system
  - o portions of many different systems that fight disease
  - o lymphatic system
  - o picks up fluids leaked from the capillaries
  - o houses white blood cells.

- cardiovascular system
  - o transports nutrients and gas waste
  - o supports immune function.

- urinary system
  - o gets rid of toxic waste out of blood
  - o regulates electrolytes, fluids, and pH balance.

- digestive system
  - o breaks down food into the building blocks for the body.

- respiratory system
  - o portions, moistens, and heats air
  - o exchanges gas.

- nervous system
  - o sensory input
  - o interprets input or thought
  - o feedback and signal responses
  - o coordinates muscles, vital functions, and reactions.

- endocrine system
  o secretes hormones that regulate growth, metabolism, and general body functions.

- reproductive system
  o produces offspring
  o produces hormones.

2. The Blood

Blood supplies food and oxygen to all the cells in our body, and the lymph takes and removes toxins resulting from the basic functions of cells, protecting the body.

Blood represents 8 per cent of the body weight and is formed from plasma, blood cells, and platelets.

a) Blood plasma represents 55 per cent of the blood's volume and is a mixture of proteins, enzymes, nutrients, wastes, hormones, and gases. Proteins (almost 500 types) have roles in clotting, defence, and transport and govern the distribution of water between the blood and tissue fluids.

Cells called macrophages in the liver, gut, spleen, lungs, and lymphatic tissues can break down plasma proteins so as to release their amino acids, which are used by other cells to synthesize new products. The proteins also help to keep the blood slightly basic at a stable pH. They do this by functioning as weak bases themselves to bind excess H^+ ions. By doing so, they remove excess H^+ from the blood, which keeps it slightly basic. Nota bene: the cancer cells like an acidic environment and can't survive in a basic one.

Blood has a pH of 7.35 to 7.45 and needs to be constant. If a pH imbalance arises, in a few minutes, your body must raise the pH to these values regardless of the situation; otherwise, life wouldn't be possible. If it has permanent acidity to neutralize, it will use the base of the body (calcium and magnesium taken directly from the bones and teeth), leading to the weakening of bone density over time, affecting the joints and muscles also.

We can help the body to regulate its acidity with different types of foods eaten. Fruits and vegetables consumed raw are less acidic. Animal proteins induce greater acidity, and the highest acidity is induced by the processed and refined foods—candies, sweets, sodas, coffee, beer, etc. But we will discuss this in a separate chapter, as the body's acid–alkaline balance is a very important factor in the development of cancer. Don't forget that cancer likes an acidic environment.

b) Blood cells include erythrocytes, also known as red blood cells (RBCs), and leukocytes, also known as white blood cells (WBCs).

Red blood cells (RBCs) have two main functions:

1. to pick up oxygen from the lungs and deliver it to tissues elsewhere
2. to pick up carbon dioxide from other tissues and unload it in the lungs.

How much oxygen your body tissues get depends on how many RBCs you have, how well they work, and how much time you spend in a well-oxygenated environment. A proportion of 95 per cent of a red cell is formed by a protein called haemoglobin, an iron-rich carrier of body gases. Radiotherapy and chemotherapy destroy the red cells together with other body cells.

Circulating erythrocytes live for about 120 days, and we have approximately 4.5 to 6.1 million cells per microlitre (cells/µl). As an RBC ages, its membrane grows increasingly fragile. Without key organelles (such as a nucleus, mitochondria, or ribosomes), RBCs cannot repair themselves. Many RBCs die in the spleen, where they are broken up and destroyed, but they are continuously created in the bone marrow from the stem cells.

White blood cells, or leukocytes, make up a small part of the blood's volume (about 1 per cent), and there are approximately 4,000 to 8,000 cells per microlitre of blood in a healthy person. The number increases during a cold or infection. They are produced in the thymus and bone marrow and can be found also in the spleen and lymph nodes. The white cells called lymphocytes are very important for our immune system. They identify and bind to foreigner viruses, bacteria, and fungi, preparing them to be removed by the other white cells called macrophages, which are usually dying in the process.

They also clean the body from 'dust' and other unwanted matter, being our most important asset in the fight with cancer and all other 'intruders'.

c) Platelets, or thrombocytes, are about one-third the size of a red blood cell and have an important role in blood clotting in collaboration with other thirteen factors. Also they are helpers of the immune system in fighting viruses and bacteria. Thrombocytes are produced in the bone marrow and have a life span of ten days. They present a peak of activation in the morning; this is the main reason why heart attacks and strokes occur mostly in the morning,

For more information on blood composition visit:

(http://www.myvmc.com/anatomy/blood-function-and-composition/; December 2014)

3. The Lymph

'The Lymph very closely resembles the plasma found in the veins: it is a mixture of about 90% water and 10% solutes such as proteins, cellular waste products, dissolved gases, and hormones. Lymph may also contain bacterial cells that are picked up from diseased tissues and the white blood cells that fight these pathogens. In late-stage cancer patients, lymph often contains cancerous cells that have metastasized from tumours and may form new tumours within the lymphatic system.

A special type of lymph, known as chyle, is produced in the digestive system as lymph absorbs triglycerides from the intestinal villi. Due to the presence of triglycerides, chyle has a milky white coloration.

Interstitial fluid is picked up by the lymphatic capillaries, which merge together into larger lymphatic vessels to carry lymph through the body. The structure of lymphatic vessels closely resembles that of veins: they both have thin walls and many check valves due to their shared function of carrying fluids under low pressure. Lymph is transported through lymphatic vessels by the skeletal muscle pump—contractions of skeletal muscles constrict the vessels to push the fluid forward.'

(http://www.innerbody.com/image/lympov.html-December 2014).

That's why we need to do physical activity to use our muscles and indirectly help the lymphatic system to circulate, especially when we fight cancer.

Lymph enters from several afferent lymph vessels in the lymph nodes, which function as filters. 'There are several hundred lymph nodes found mostly throughout the thorax and abdomen of the body with the highest concentrations in the axillary (armpit) and inguinal (groin) regions. The reticular fibres of the lymph node act as a net to catch any debris or cells that are present in the lymph. Macrophages and lymphocytes attack and kill any microbes caught in the reticular fibres. Efferent lymph vessels then carry the filtered lymph out of the lymph node and towards the lymphatic ducts.' It is very important to keep your lymph nodes, and do not let the surgeons take them out if you have an operation for cancer.

'Outside of the system of lymphatic vessels and lymph nodes, there are masses of non-encapsulated lymphatic tissue known as lymphatic nodules. The lymphatic nodules are associated with the mucous membranes of the body, where they work to protect the body from pathogens entering the body through open body cavities [tonsils, spleen, Peyer's patches, and thymus].'

(http://www.innerbody.com/image/lympov.html-December 2014)

To protect itself from infection from an endless supply of pathogens, the body employs many different types of immunity: fever, inflammation, natural killer cells, body secretions, and phagocytes. All cells communicate between them via chemicals and electrical impulses in order to maintain a balance suitable for their perfect functioning.

I said earlier that blood supplies and is in constant contact with all cells in our body, and it needs to have a constant pH of 7.35–7.45.

The normal state of our cells is an alkaline one. In an aerobic state (with oxygen), each cell produces its energy through the mitochondria, also called power plants, because they contain oxidation–reduction enzymes needed in breathing. Respiration produces energy for organisms, and this energy is stored in ATP molecules. Mitochondria have their own genetic material, the mitochondrial DNA, which contains the genetic information needed for synthesis of respiratory enzymes; here, the oxygen, glucose, and fructose are essential!

Now imagine that, to escape the daily acidity excesses, the blood throws it to the cells. The healthy cells become highly acidic with very low oxygen content. Now they have only two options: either to die or to transform. Usually they transform and become a cell adapted to an oxygen-free environment, learning to live in an anaerobic environment and producing energy by fermentation. This is the cancer cell. And this should not scare us; all of us have between 1,000 and 10,000 cancer cells every day in our body.

The immune system and white blood cells destroy them. In this case, the question is, why then does cancer do such great havoc? Why is our own immune system not protecting us from cancer?

Here's the interesting part—the intelligence of the cells.

The cells which become cancerous know they will be decimated by white blood cells and have found a way to make themselves invisible to the immune system. They wrap themselves with some normal and healthy cells (trophoblasts), which is a kind of wolf in lamb's skin, and thus, the immune system does not see what's inside.

It's the exact the same thing we have met before in nature. A foetus in its mother's body is composed of chromosomes from both parents. If the mother's immune system sees it, it would attack immediately. In 1902, John Beard, a professor of embryology at the University of Edinburgh, Scotland, wrote an article published in the medical journal *The Lancet*, which stated that between cancer cells and some pre-embryonal cells characteristic to the initial phase of pregnancy, there is no difference.

'Stem cells are some cells that can form whatever. In this case, 80 per cent of them are in the ovary and testes (to create life), and 20 per cent are in the remaining part of the body to regenerate any kind of tissue in the event of an accident.

Beard noted that the placenta (which is actually composed of trophoblast cells) looks almost identical to cancer cells. The placenta has an exploding growth during the first three months of pregnancy and then slows down growing. Why?

The child's pancreas starts to work after the third month of pregnancy, producing an enzyme called trypsin. And it seems that this enzyme stops placental growth. By the ninth month, placental growth is very slow because in the foetus, a new pancreas is already working at full capacity and then, together with the maternal pancreas, produces this enzyme in quantities large enough to pierce the placenta. Once the placenta is punched out, the amniotic fluid (water) breaks, and the immune system sees what is 'hidden' there, immediately triggering travail; basically, it pushes out the 'parasite'.

Trypsin, apart from digesting the trophoblast cells (placenta), digests animal protein too in our daily diet. The high-protein diet, which some of us have, need large amounts of trypsin to digest food three times a day. The pancreas, which produces trypsin, also becomes weak, and it does not produce any sufficient trypsin for the digestion. If we have cancer, it can't destroy the coating of the cancer cells, which have been hiding them from the immune system.' (http://www.scribd.com/doc/205106778/Daca-Ai-Inteles-Acest-Articol-Ti-Ai-Salvat-Singur-Viata#scribd- December 2014)

That's why it is important to reduce the animal protein intake if diagnosed with cancer. By doing so, we help the body to keep the trypsin in higher quantity to send it to destroy the cancerous cells' membranes so the immune system can attack them.

If we do not eat anything of animal origin, all available trypsin will digest and uncover the cancer cells to make these visible to white blood cells, and they will be able to fulfil their role.

Chemotherapy and radiation will kill cancer cells; however, these will kill healthy cells too and paralyzes white blood cells! After the first session of chemotherapy, they become unable to fight, and we cannot rely on the immune system any more, losing our most important ally.

So our body has all the necessary equipment to fight cancer, and all that we need to do is to understand those mechanisms and to help them in their job. We need to learn what tools to use, what plants have the power to heal, and how to combine different healing techniques.

There are foods and plant extracts which can destroy the tumourous cells without destroying the healthy cells in the body, and I will present most of them in this book.

Cancer

Cancer is defined as a development of abnormal cells that divide uncontrollably and have the ability to infiltrate and destroy normal body tissue.

The question is, why do those cells start acting chaotic? What is the cause?

We will try to get the answer in this chapter.

In order to defeat cancer, let's learn a bit about it. Let's know our enemy, its likes and dislikes, so we can make a strategic plan of attack!

Cancers are classified in two ways: by the type of tissue in which the cancer originates (histological type) and by primary site, the location in the body where the cancer first developed.

The following classification and description was collected from http://training.seer.cancer.gov (December 2014).

> From a histological standpoint there are hundreds of different cancers, which are grouped into six major categories:
>
> - Carcinoma
> - Sarcoma
> - Myeloma
> - Leukemia
> - Lymphoma
> - Mixed Types.

Carcinoma

Carcinoma refers to a malignant neoplasm of epithelial origin or cancer of the internal or external lining of the body. Carcinomas, malignancies of epithelial tissue, account for 80 to 90 percent of all cancer cases.

Epithelial tissue is found throughout the body. It is present in the skin, as well as the covering and lining of organs and internal passageways, such as the gastrointestinal tract.

Carcinomas are divided into two major subtypes: adenocarcinoma, which develops in an organ or gland, and squamous cell carcinoma, which originates in the squamous epithelium.

Adenocarcinomas generally occur in mucus membranes and are first seen as a thickened plaque-like white mucosa. They often spread easily through the soft tissue where they occur. Squamous cell carcinomas occur in many areas of the body.

Most carcinomas affect organs or glands capable of secretion, such as the breasts, or the lungs, colon, prostate or bladder.

Sarcoma

Sarcoma refers to cancer that originates in supportive and connective tissues such as bones, tendons, cartilage, muscle, and fat. Generally occurring in young adults, the most common sarcoma often develops as a painful mass on the bone. Sarcoma tumors usually resemble the tissue in which they grow.

Examples of sarcomas are:

- Osteosarcoma or osteogenic sarcoma (bone)
- Chondrosarcoma (cartilage)
- Leiomyosarcoma (smooth muscle)
- Rhabdomyosarcoma (skeletal muscle)
- Mesothelial sarcoma or mesothelioma (membranous lining of body cavities)
- Fibrosarcoma (fibrous tissue)
- Angiosarcoma or hemangioendothelioma (blood vessels)
- Liposarcoma (adipose tissue)
- Glioma or astrocytoma (neurogenic connective tissue found in the brain)
- Myxosarcoma (primitive embryonic connective tissue)
- Mesenchymous or mixed mesodermal tumor (mixed connective tissue types).

Myeloma

Myeloma is cancer that originates in the plasma cells of bone marrow. The plasma cells produce some of the proteins found in blood.

Leukaemia

Leukaemia ('liquid cancers' or 'blood cancers') are cancers of the bone marrow (the site of blood cell production). The word leukaemia means 'white blood' in Greek. The disease is often associated with the overproduction of immature white blood cells. These immature white blood cells do not perform as well as they should, therefore the patient is often prone to infection. Leukaemia also affects red blood cells and can cause poor blood clotting and fatigue due to anaemia.

Lymphoma

Lymphomas develop in the glands or nodes of the lymphatic system, a network of vessels, nodes, and organs (specifically the spleen, tonsils, and thymus) that purify bodily fluids and produce infection-fighting white blood cells, or lymphocytes. See more information about the Lymphatic system at the beginning of this chapter. Unlike the leukaemia which are sometimes called 'liquid cancers,' lymphomas are 'solid cancers.' Lymphomas may also occur in specific organs such as the stomach, breast or brain. These lymphomas are referred to as extra nodal lymphomas. The lymphomas are sub classified into two categories: Hodgkin lymphoma and Non-Hodgkin lymphoma.

Mixed Types

The mixed type components may be within one category or from different categories. Some examples are:

- adenosquamous carcinoma
- mixed mesodermal tumor
- carcinosarcoma
- teratocarcinoma.

For more information about cancer classification, go to http://training.seer.cancer.gov/disease/categories/classification.html.

Based on metastatic potential, there are two classifications of cancers:

(a) benign tumours—when neoplastic growth remains clustered as a single mass
(b) malignant tumours—when tumour invades normal tissue and spreads throughout the body.

It is estimated that human body consists of 100 trillion cells. Almost all of these cells get turned over within approximately 100 days, thus suggesting an apoptosis/cell death rate of 100–130 billion cells each day. What is the mechanism of this mode of cell death in normal cells is unclear and it is maybe connected with the hidden 'intelligence of the Universe' which we, humans are not able to understand yet.

Every person has cancer cells in the body. These cancer cells do not show up in the standard tests until they have multiplied to a few million.

Cancer cells occur between 6 to more than 10 times in a person's lifetime.'

(http://www.truthorfiction.com/rumors/j/johnshop
kinscancer.htm-March 2015)

It seems that cancer cells need to divide and multiply ten years for them to be seen by medical devices and be diagnosed as cancer in phase I.

> When the person's immune system is strong the cancer cells will be destroyed and prevented from multiplying and forming tumors.

> When a person has cancer it indicates that the person has nutritional deficiencies which alliterated his immune system. These could be due to genetic, but also to environmental, food and lifestyle factors.

> To overcome the multiple nutritional deficiencies, changing diet to eat more adequately and healthy, 4–5 times/day and by including supplements will strengthen the immune system.

> Chemotherapy involves poisoning the rapidly-growing cancer cells but also destroys rapidly-growing healthy cells in the bone marrow and can cause organ damage, like liver, kidneys, heart, lungs etc., disturbing the whole normal function of the body. Radiation while destroying cancer cells also burns, scars and damages healthy cells, tissues and organs.

> Initial treatment with chemotherapy and radiation will often reduce tumor size. However prolonged use of chemotherapy and radiation do not result in more tumor destruction.

> When the body has too much toxic burden from chemotherapy and radiation the immune system is either compromised or destroyed, hence the person can succumb to various kinds of infections and

complications. Chemotherapy and radiation can cause cancer cells to mutate and become resistant and difficult to destroy. Surgery can also cause cancer cells to spread to other sites.

Rapidly growing tumor cells exhibit rates of glycolysis up to 200 times higher than those of healthy cells. The cancer cells has 96 receptors for sugar comparative with a normal cell which has only 4. The energy produced is used to fuel the growth and spread of cancer. So if you wish to starve the cancer cell, avoid the sugar and all the sweets or artificial sweeteners.

On the other hand, healthy cells do not primarily use glycolysis for energy production, because it's an inefficient way to produce energy. Instead, healthy cells use oxygen to produce energy from glucose in the mitochondria (the metabolic center) of the cell. The switch to glycolysis as an energy source occurs when cells of a tumor (either benign or pre-cancerous) become deprived of oxygen in their environment.

As a result, their mitochondria cannot work properly. These abnormal cells then 'switch off' their mitochondria. Mitochondria are essential to the process of inducing apoptosis (the process by which abnormal cells self-destruct). When cells switch off mitochondria, they develop 'immorality' and will continue to divide becoming cancer.

An effective way to battle cancer is to starve the cancer cells by not feeding it with the foods it needs to grow and multiply.' (http://www.truthorfiction.com/rumors/j/johnshopkinscancer.htm;March 2015).

Let's see what cancer feeds on!

Cancer cells feed on:

- Sugar and sugar substitutes—like NutraSweet, Equal, Spoonful, etc.—are made with aspartame, and they are harmful. 'A better natural substitute would be Manuka honey or Stevia, but only in very small amounts. Table salt has a chemical added to make it white in colour. Better alternative is Bragg's aminos, Himalayan salt or sea salt.' (http://www.truthorfiction.com/rumors/j/johnshopkinscancer. htm ;March 2015).

- Milk and dairy products are acidic and can cause the body to produce mucus, especially in the gastrointestinal tract. 'By cutting off milk and substituting it with unsweetened soy milk, cancer cells are being starved. Also milk can contain all the hormones, medicines and chemicals given to the caws to increase the production. Yogurt has good bacteria in it which help the digestive system, so time to time you can have it especially if it is organic and with no sugar or fruits added.'(http://www.truthorfiction.com/rumors/j/john shopkinscancer.htm;March 2015).

- Meat. Cancer cells thrive in an acidic environment. A meat-based diet is acidic, so it is best to eat fish and other meat, like chicken and seafood. 'Meat also contains livestock antibiotics, growth hormones and parasites, which are all harmful, especially to people with cancer. Meat protein is difficult to digest and requires a lot of digestive enzymes. Undigested meat remaining in the intestines becomes putrefied and leads to more toxic build up. Cancer cell walls have a tough protein covering. By refraining from or eating less meat it frees more enzymes like Trypsine, (presented above), to attack the protein walls of cancer cells and allows the body's killer cells to destroy the cancer cells.' (.http://www.truthorfiction.com/rumors/j/johnshopkins cancer.htm-March 2015)

A diet made of 80% fresh vegetables and juice, whole grains, seeds, nuts and a little fruits help put the body into an alkaline environment. Fresh vegetable juices provide live enzymes that are easily absorbed and reach down to cellular levels within 15 minutes to nourish and enhance growth of healthy cells. To obtain live enzymes for building healthy cells try and drink fresh vegetable juice (most vegetables including bean sprouts) and eat some raw vegetables 2 or 3 times a day. Enzymes are destroyed at temperatures of 104 degrees F (40 degrees C), so avoid cooking.

Some supplements build up the immune system (IP6, Essiac, anti-oxidants, Astragalus, Echinaceea, vitamins, minerals, EFAs etc.) to enable the body's own killer cells to destroy cancer cells. Other supplements like vitamin E are known to cause apoptosis, or programmed cell death, the body's normal method of disposing of damaged, unwanted, or unneeded cells.

Cancer is a disease of the mind, body, and spirit. A proactive and positive spirit will help the cancer warrior be a survivor. Anger, un-forgiveness and bitterness put the body into a stressful and acidic environment. Learn to have a positive, loving and forgiving spirit. Learn to relax and enjoy life.

Cancer cells cannot thrive in an oxygenated environment. Exercising daily, and deep breathing help to get more oxygen down to the cellular level. Oxygen therapy is another means employed to destroy cancer cells. (http://www.truthorfiction.com/rumors/j/johnshopkinscancer.htm, March 2015)

Apoptosis

The ability of tumor cell populations to expand in number is determined not only by the rate of cell proliferation but also by the rate of cell death. Apoptosis is a major source of cell death, thus agents that trigger apoptosis/cell death, could be the most promising candidates as therapeutic for cancer.

There are two major pathways of cell death, apoptosis (death by suicide) and necrosis (death by injury). Apoptosis is also known as programmed cell death and involves a series of biochemical events leading to characteristic cell morphology alteration and death. Necrosis is caused by external factors, such as infection, toxins, or trauma.

Apoptosis is a normal physiological process that is required for the maintenance of cell homeostasis. The cellular changes involved in this process are both morphological and biochemical, including disintegration of the cytoskeleton and subsequent cell shrinkage, chromatin condensation, and activation of specific proteases, called caspases.

Apoptosis can be initiated by a variety of internal and external stimuli, including receptor ligation and toxic insults. Apoptosis not only plays a crucial role in tissue development and homeostasis, but is also involved in a wide range of pathological conditions. Apoptotic cell death is accompanied by a series of complex biochemical events and definite morphologic changes, which include cell shrinkage, chromatin condensation, DNA fragmentation, membrane budding, and the appearance of membrane-associated apoptotic bodies. Failure to accurately undergo apoptosis can cause severe anomalies, ranging from autoimmune disease to cancer.'

(http://www.ncbi.nlm.nih.gov/pmc/articles/PMC211
7903/;December 2014)

There are several natural products which can induce apoptosis and
cancer remission.

1. Curcumin

Curcumin is a natural diphenolic compound derived from turmeric
(*Curcuma longa*) and has proven to be a modulator of intracellular
signalling pathways that control cancer cell growth, inflammation,
invasion, apoptosis and cell death, which reveals its anticancer potential.

Curcumin has a diverse range of molecular targets,
supporting the concept that it acts upon numerous
biochemical and molecular cascades. Curcumin
physically binds to as many as 33 different proteins,
including thioredoxin reductase, cyclooxygenase-2,
(COX2), protein kinase C, 5-lipoxygenase (5-LOX),
and tubulin. Various molecular targets modulated by
this agent include transcription factors, growth factors
and their receptors, cytokines, enzymes, and genes
regulating cell proliferation, and apoptosis. Curcumin
has been shown to inhibit the proliferation and survival
of almost all types of tumor cells. Accumulating
evidence suggests that the mode of curcumin-induced
cell death is mediated both by the activation of cell death
pathways and by the inhibition of growth/proliferation
pathways. Many studies indicate the selective role
of curcumin towards cancer cells than normal cells.
Because curcumin mediates its effect through multiple
cell signalling pathways, the likelihood of developing
resistance to it is less. (http://www.ncbi.nlm.nih.gov/
pmc/articles/PMC2758121/)

2. Iscador (Mistletoe)

Viscum album or mistletoe is a semiparasitic plant that grows on apple, pine, oak, and other trees in Europe and Asia. Mistletoe is shrouded in mystery. *Truizis* (Celtic priests) considered it a sacred plant, a panacea that can remove all bad things, and it was collected with golden knives in special ceremonies. Old medical herbalists used it as an excellent medicine for combating epilepsy, hysteria, chronic spasms, and heart problems. In the beginning of the twentieth century, Rudolf Steiner pioneered the use of mistletoe therapy in connection to the treatment of cancer.

The benefits of the mistletoe treatment are:

    a.   stimulates the immune system
    b.   inhibits the growth of cancer cells
    c.   reduces the size of tumours
    d.   improves the quality of life
    e.   lessens the pain associated with tumours
    f.   improves the ability to cope with radiotherapy and chemotherapy
    g.   lifts depressive mood.

The leaves and stems are collected only from early October until mid December and then in March and April. In other months, *Viscum* has no healing power.

One of the most known company which produces *Viscum* extract under the name of Iscador, Helixor, Eurixor, and Isorel, most of which are available in Europe, is Weleda.

In Australia, you can get it from New Zealand through the Melbourne Therapy Centre; address 221 Wonga Rd, Warranwood VIC 3134;tel. (03) 9876 3011 ; www.**melbournetherapy**.org.au/

Used in cancer treatment for over 90 years, mistletoe therapy has been widely researched and is still subject to ongoing development. It is one of the most frequently prescribed complementary treatments for cancer in central Europe. There it is available in GP practices, specialist cancer centres, and hospitals.

Mistletoe therapy can be given in a variety of ways:

- injection under the skin (subcutaneous)
- infusion through a drip (intravenous)
- injection into the tumour (intratumour)
- orally (by mouth).

The treatment need to be done for months or years depending on the stage of cancer.

Mistletoe contains a few immunostimulatory and cytotoxic proteins, lectins, and polypeptides, which slow and regress the tumour growth by inducing apoptosis, increase the natural killer cell activity, and protect the DNA during the chemotherapy.

Mistletoe treatment has very few side effects, including allergic reactions, local pain, or rare nausea symptoms.

To avoid potential interactions, be sure to let your health-care provider know if you're using this or any other type of complementary therapy. Always take under the advice and supervision of a health practitioner.

For research or books on Iscador (mistletoe), go to Lukas Clinic's website (http://www.lukasklinik.ch/English/Default1.htm).

For Australia, go to Melbourne Therapy Clinic (http://melbournetherapy. org.au/).

They use these products in their treatment programs.

You can also go to the following:

http://www.totnescancerhealthcentre.com/?p=7912

www.sph.uth.tmc.edu/utcam/summary/mistletoe.htm

http://commonweal.org/herbs.html

http://alternativecancertreatmentgerson.com/iscador-therapy/

http://www.cancure.org/iscador_mistletoe.htm.

3. Resveratrol

> The polyphenolic compound Resveratrol is a naturally occurring phytochemical and can be found in many plant species, including grapes, peanuts and various herbs. Several studies have established that Resveratrol can exert anti-oxidant and anti-inflammatory activities. It also has activity in the regulation of multiple cellular events associated with carcinogenesis, properties in relationship to oestrogen, effect on lipid metabolism, cardiovascular effects, and role on gene expression. Resveratrol has also been examined in several model systems for its potential effect against cancer. Its anti-cancer effects include its role as a chemo preventive agent, its ability to inhibit cell proliferation, its direct effect in cytotoxicity by induction of apoptosis and on its potential therapeutic effect in pre-clinical studies. In addition, Resveratrol has been shown to exert sensitization effects on cancer cells that will result in a synergistic cytotoxic activity when Resveratrol is used in combination with other cytotoxic drugs in drug-resistant tumour cells. (http://www.ncbi.nlm.nih.gov/pmc/articles/PMC4013237/)

4. Caffeic Acid Phenethyl Ester in Propolis (Alternative Name: CAPE)

Propolis is a resinous mixture that bees collect from tree buds, sap flows, or other botanical sources. It is used as a sealant for unwanted open spaces in the hive. Propolis is used for small gaps (approximately 6 millimetres or 0.24 inches), and it is chemically different from the beeswax, which is used for bigger gaps. Its colour varies depending on its botanical source, and the most common is dark brown. Propolis is sticky at and above room temperature, at 20 degrees Celsius (68 degrees Fahrenheit).

> The composition of propolis varies from hive to hive, from district to district, and from season to season. Normally it is dark brown in colour, but it can be found in green, red, black, and white, depending on the sources of the resin found in the particular hive area. Honey bees are opportunists, gathering what they need from available sources, and detailed analyses show that the chemical composition of propolis varies considerably from region to region, along with the vegetation. In northern temperate climates, for example, bees collect resins from herbs and trees, like conifers and poplars. (The biological role of resin in trees is to seal wounds and defend against bacteria, fungi and insects.) 'Typical' northern temperate propolis has approximately 50 constituents, primarily resins and vegetable balsams (50%), waxes (30%), essential oils (10%), and pollen (5%). In Neotropical regions, in addition to a large variety of trees, bees may also gather resin from flowers in the genera *Clusia* and *Dalechampia*, which are the only known plant genera that produce floral resins to attract pollinators.((http://en.wikipedia.org/wiki/Propolis; December 2014)

The following are the substances that give propolis its healing properties:

- 55 per cent resinous compounds and balsam
- 30 per cent beeswax
- 10 per cent ethereal and aromatic oils
- 5 per cent bee pollen.

Propolis contains many minerals, including magnesium, calcium, phosphorus, potassium, beta carotene, bioflavonoids, vitamins B_1 and B_2, pinobanksin-5-methylether, galangin, chrysin, pinobanksin, pinocembrin, cinnamic acid, cinnamyl alcohol, vanillin, tetochrysin, isalpinin, and ferulic acid.

Galangin and chrysin are important oestrogen and testosterone regulators; this is possibly the reason why it is used to treat hormonal conditions for men and women. Caffeic acid is anti-inflammatory, anti-oxidation, anticancer, antibacterial, antiviral, antifungal, and has immunomodulatory effects.

A professional beekeeper told me that he has problems collecting propolis in Australia because of the production being far lesser (due to the lack on resinous trees and plants) than in Romania, where he was living before. But there is a good source of propolis in New Zealand that has a high concentration of caffeic acid phenethyl ester (CAPE).

CAPE (3-(3,4-dihydroxyphenyl)-2-propenoic acid 2-phenylethyl ester) is an antioxidant; it is also antimitogenic, anticarcinogenic, anti-inflammatory, and antiviral. It inhibits the growth of breast cancer cells and breast cancer stem cells, induces cell cycle arrest and apoptosis, and suppresses angiogenesis. Gene arrays show that CAPE causes extensive changes in gene expression in both ER+ and ER– types of breast cancer cells, including the inhibition of NF-κB. It also suppresses lipid peroxidation and inhibits ornithine decarboxylase, protein tyrosine kinase, and lipoxygenase activities.

> As a concentrated source of bioflavonoids, (it contains more bioflavonoids than oranges), propolis may help strengthen capillary walls and connective tissue, enhance absorption of vitamin C, and play a supportive role in reducing respiratory infections, bleeding gums, varicose veins, cancer and many other ailments.

(www.bee-pollen-buzz.com/bee-propolis.html- March 2015)

For more info, see the following:

http://www.bee-pollen-buzz.com/bee-propolis-health-benefits.html

http://www.bee-pollen-buzz.com/what-is-bee-propolis.html).

http://en.wikipedia.org/wiki/Propolis.

5. Vitamin B$_{17}$ (Laetrile)

> Laetrile (i.e. amygdalin or Vitamin B17) therapy is one of the most popular and best known alternative cancer treatments. It is very simple to use and is very effective if used in high enough doses and if the product is of high quality and if it is combined with an effective cancer diet and key supplements (in other words, you need to do your homework to maximize its benefits).

> The Dr. Philip Binzel list of foods that contain laetrile include: apricot kernels, peach kernels, grape seeds, blackberries, blueberries, strawberries, bean sprouts, lima beans and macadamia nuts (to name but a few).

> Other things rich in laetrile are millet grain and buckwheat grain. Breads made with these grains, however, generally do not contain a high percentage of millet or buckwheat or else they would be too hard.

> Also, the seeds of berry plants, such as red raspberries and black raspberries are rich in laetrile. Red raspberries also have a second cancer killer in their seeds: Ellagic Acid, a phenolic. About four dozen foods have Ellagic Acid, but Red Raspberries have the highest concentration. Strawberries also have Ellagic Acid.

> Basically, the seeds of any fruit, except citrus fruits, have laetrile.

Of course, apricot kernels are the best source of laetrile. Those who do not yet have cancer might want to plant a few apricot or peach trees in their back yard for a long term source of laetrile. The kernels can be frozen while still in the shell.

If you search for 'apricot kernels' (use the quotes) on Google you will be able to find a lot of vendors of apricot kernels. Be advised, however, that apricot kernel sites cannot legally make any medical claims about laetrile being used to treat cancer.

Laetrile works by targeting and killing cancer cells and building the immune system to fend off future outbreaks of cancer. It uses two different methods for killing cancer cells. It involves a strict diet (as do all cancer treatments) and several supplements.

Most experts will recommend a **daily** dose of apricot kernels from between 24 kernels a day up to 40 kernels a day, spread throughout the day. For a person in remission, 16 apricot kernels a day should be used as a minimum. The FDA claims that laetrile is toxic. This is an absolute lie. Read the first chapter of Alive and Well by Dr. Philip E Binzel (http://www.whale.to/m/binzel.html) to see how absurd the FDA claim is. It is only toxic to cancer cells.

The FDA has made the purchase of laetrile supplements almost impossible to obtain, even though it is a perfectly natural and safe supplement. In order for a doctor to use laetrile supplements, they or their patient must 'confess' to the FDA that the doctor is using laetrile in their practice. In other words, laetrile supplements are effectively illegal because no doctor wants to admit they are using laetrile.

Fortunately they are available over the Internet either as apricot kernels or pills and in some cases in liquid form.' (http://www.cancertutor.com/laetrile/; March 2015).

I ordered them on this website: www.tjsupply.com. TJ Supply's address is 416 W. San Ysidro Blvd, Ste L447, San Ysidro, California 92173. USA number is (619) 819 7531. Toll-free number is 888-281-6663. Email is b17@tjsupply.com.

They will tell you how to get the FDA approval.

> Most people take laetrile in the form of apricot kernels. In the middle of a peach or apricot is a hard shell. If you break open the hard shell with a 'nut cracker', pliers or hammer, you will find a small seed/kernel in the middle that looks like an almond. However, it is much softer than an almond and certainly does not taste like an almond. It is this seed that is rich in natural laetrile.

If you obtain laetrile **pills,** it is important to take them with natural water during a meal. (http://www.cancertutor.com/laetrile/;March 2015).

How does laetrile work?

> 'When the laetrile compound molecule comes across a cancer cell, it is broken down into 2 molecules of glucose, 1 molecule of hydrogen cyanide and 1 molecule of benzaldehyde. In the early days of laetrile research it was assumed that the hydrogen cyanide molecule was the major cancer cell killing molecule, but now it is known that it is the benzaldehyde molecule that is by far the major reason the cancer cell is killed.

> The reason laetrile therapy takes so long to work, in spite of the marvelous design of the laetrile molecule, is

because if the laetrile molecule happens to chemically react with the enzyme of a non-cancerous cell (i.e. rhodanese), before it reacts with the enzyme of a cancerous cell (beta-glucosidase), the rhodanese will break apart the laetrile molecule in such a way that it can no longer kill a cancer cell. Thus you have to take enough laetrile molecules, over a long enough time, that enough laetrile molecules coincidently (as far as we know) hits all of the cancer cells first.

The second way that laetrile therapy works is because of the laetrile diet. Like the metabolic diet, it is designed to build up the trypsin and chymotrypsin in the body, and let them work on the cancer cells. What they do is break down the enzymes surrounding the cancer cell so the white blood cells can identify and kill the cancer cell.

One of the good side-effects of laetrile therapy is that more Vitamin B12 is made in the body'.(http://www.cancertutor.com/laetrile/;March 2015).

First, make sure you supplement laetrile therapy with Vitamin C. Vitamin C and Vitamin B_{12} are by themselves treatments for cancer.

Second, make sure you get the nutrients necessary for laetrile to work:

- zinc (the transport mechanism for laetrile)
- vitamin C (build up to 6 grams a day)
- manganese
- magnesium
- selenium
- vitamins B_6, B_9, and B_{12}
- vitamin A
- vitamin E (at least 2,000 international units).

Also, during the laetrile therapy, it is *critical* to take the pancreatic or proteolytic enzymes! The most common is Megazyme Forte, which contains trypsin, chymotrypsin, bromelain. Two pills should be taken three times a day.

> Other pancreatic enzymes (also known as proteolytic enzymes) are: Vitalzym, 10Zymes (also from Essense of Life), and Wobenzym N.

> However, note that they are blood thinners and should be taken within the vendor's recommended maximum dosage (on the bottle). These are critical for the laetrile molecules to work at peak efficiency.

> Note that zinc is also one of the most critical parts of this therapy:

> *'Zinc is the transportation mechanism for laetrile and nitrilosides in the body. Biochemists and researchers have found that you can give Laetrile to a patient until its coming out of the ears of the patient, but, if that patient did not have sufficient level of Zinc, none of the laetrile would get into the tissues of the body. They also found that nothing heals within the body without sufficient vitamin C. They also found that magnesium; selenium, vitamin A, and B all played an important part in maintaining the body's defence mechanism. This is why its important to understand that cancer is best treated with a total nutritional program consisting of diet, vitamins, minerals, laetrile and pancreatic enzymes'.* (http://www.thefountainoflife.ws/ cancer/zinc.htm) (Dec-2014)_http://www. cancertutor.com/laetrile/

6. Vitamin C Intravenous

Vitamin C (ascorbic acid) can be taken orally or intravenously.

> Orally, start taking a low dosage of vitamin C every day
> (about 500 to 1000 MG) and slowly build your way up
> to 10,000 to 25,000 MG per day. This will take some
> time to get your body used to such levels so don't be too
> anxious about getting to the higher dosages right away.
> Some symptoms of too high a dose could be headaches,
> nausea, diarrhoea, etc. This does not mean that the
> product is not working. On the contrary, it means that
> your body is being detoxified too fast so you need to
> back off on the dosage. You want to detox your body
> at a slow rate so you won't get the symptoms described
> above'.(http://www.1cure4cancer.com/continue_pp2.
> htm ; March 2015).

'Ascorbate is processed by the body in different ways when administered
orally versus intravenous mode of administration,' says Heidi Ledford
in *Nature* magazine, and the difference is usually misunderstood. 'Oral
doses of vitamin C act as antioxidants, protecting cells from damage
caused by reactive oxygen-containing compounds. But intravenous
vitamin C may have the opposite effect, by encouraging the formation
of one of these compounds: hydrogen peroxide. And the cancer cells are
particularly susceptible to damage as they are compounds containing
reactive oxygen.

> When delivered in a 'drip', much higher concentrations
> of C can be attained. At these higher concentrations,
> vitamin C has different characteristics than if given
> orally. While oral vitamin C boosts immunity and
> assists tissue repair, it is too weak to do much to kill
> or inhibit cancer cells. But at high doses delivered
> directly into the bloodstream, it may act to increase
> levels of hydrogen peroxide deep in the tissues where
> cancer cells lurk. Peroxide-mediated killing is one of

the white blood cells' key mechanisms for fighting infection and cancer.

Research currently under way has shown that high concentrations of vitamin C can stop the growth or even kill a wide range of cancer cells. Only intravenous administration of vitamin C can deliver the high doses found to be effective against cancer.

IV vitamin C, when administered by a trained, experienced physician, is safe and well-tolerated, even at doses as high as 100,000 mg (100 grams) per day. Proper blood tests must be done to ensure that it is well-tolerated, and the patient must be monitored. Doses must be gradually adjusted upward. Not all patients are candidates for IV vitamin C. Vitamin C can be safely administered even while patients are undergoing chemo and radiation.

Intravenous vitamin C remains one of the key in support of recovery from cancer, and it is hoped that additional research, now under way, will further document its benefits'.(http://drhoffman.com/article/intravenous-vitamin-c-for-cancer-2/ ;March 2015).

There are many private clinics and naturopaths in Australia administrating intravenous Vitamin C.

In Melbourne, I know (and used) two big clinics:

a. National Institute of Integrative Medicine (NIIM)
    21 Burwood Rd, Hawthorn, VIC 3122
    (03) 9804 0646

b. Melbourne Therapy Centre
    221 Wonga Rd, Warranwood, VIC 3134
    (03) 9876 3011

See more at the following:

http://viataverdeviu.ro/studiuinjectiile-cu-doze-mari-de-vitamina-c-anihileaza-cancerul/

http://drhoffman.com/article/intravenous-vitamin-c-for-cancer-2/.

7. DMSO/MMS

'Dimethyl sulfoxide (C_2H_6OS), or DMSO, is a sulfur-containing organic compound. DMSO occurs naturally in vegetables, fruits grains, and animal products. DMSO was first synthesized in 1866 as a by-product of paper manufacturing. Therapeutic interest began in 1963. DMSO was reported to penetrate through the skin and produce analgesia, decrease pain, and promote tissue healing. DMSO is available for both non-medicinal and medicinal uses. The major clinical use of DMSO is to relieve symptoms of interstitial cystitis.(http://www.health-matrix.net/2011/03/15/dmso-the-real-miracle-solution/-March2015)

DMSO is a prescription medicine and dietary supplement. It can be taken by mouth, applied to the skin (used topically), or injected into the veins (used intravenously or by IV).

DMSO is taken by mouth, used topically, or given intravenously for the management of amyloidosis and related symptoms. Amyloidosis is a condition in which certain proteins are deposited abnormally in organs and tissues.

DMSO is used topically to decrease pain and speed the healing of wounds, burns, and muscle and skeletal injuries. DMSO is also used topically to treat painful conditions such as headache, inflammation, osteoarthritis, rheumatoid arthritis, and severe facial pain called tic douloureux. It is used topically for foot conditions including bunions, calluses, and fungus on toenails; and for skin conditions including keloid scars and scleroderma. It is sometimes used topically to treat skin and tissue damage caused by chemotherapy when it leaks from the IV that is used to deliver it. DMSO is used either alone or in combination with a drug called idoxuridine to treat pain associated with shingles (herpes zoster infection).

Intravenously, DMSO is used to lower abnormally high blood pressure in the brain. It is also given intravenously to treat bladder infections (interstitial cystitis) and chronic inflammatory bladder disease. The U. S. Food and Drug Administration (FDA) has approved certain DMSO products for placement inside the bladder to treat symptoms of chronic inflammatory bladder disease. DMSO is sometimes placed inside bile ducts with other medications to treat bile duct stones.'(http://www.health-matrix.net/2011/03/15/dmso-the-real-miracle-solution/; March 2015)

Remember that DMSO is a carrier, and you can add to it any of the substances presented above, or any other substance you may know that can treat cancer!

If you choose to combine it with chlorine dioxide (sodium chlorite plus citric acid), note that the chlorine dioxide must be made *fresh* every hour because chlorine dioxide is a gas and is only stable in liquids for about half an hour.

(Note: '1 drop' of chlorine dioxide is made from 1 drop of sodium chlorite (i.e. MMS—Miracle Mineral Supplement) and 1 drop of citric acid)

For this protocol the amount of chlorine dioxide (measured in 'drops') can build-up to 10 drops an hour, or more. The goal is to get to 10 drops an hour, six time a day.

Do not increase the dosage if the skin can no longer tolerate it (after using multiple locations on the skin), and you should drop this down to a dose that the skin can tolerate.

However, the good news is that the DMSO can be put anywhere on the skin of the body. For example, even if the cancer is in the liver, the DMSO can be put on the legs or arms.

Of course, you start putting the DMSO as close to the cancer as possible, but as the skin complains, start moving the DMSO away from the original spot.

DMSO cream or MSM cream can be purchased at a health food store and can be used after the DMSO has penetrated the skin completely to help the skin. '(http://www.health-matrix.net/2011/03/15/ dmso-the-real-miracle-solution/-March2015)

As I said, it is the best cancer treatment because DMSO targets the cancer cells and the chlorine dioxide kills the cancer cells so they revert into normal cells. DMSO and chlorine dioxide actually bind together so most of the chlorine dioxide actually ends up inside the cancer cells

I used DMSO only on the skin on topic applications (without chlorine, but I took MSM orally) in the painful areas (joints, bones), and it was very effective after the radiation treatment, but I didn't use it internally.

Please consult your doctor/naturopath before starting this treatment.

The above information about DMSO, was collected from the article 'DMSO: The Real Miracle Solution' found on http://www.health-matrix.net/2011/03/15/dmso-the-real-miracle-solution/.

For more info, go to the following:

http://www.new-cancer-treatments.org/Cancer/DMSO_CD.html

http://www.natmedtalk.com/showthread.php?t=4491

http://www.healthline.com/natstandardcontent/dmso.

8. Tetrahydrocannabinol(THC) and Cannabidiol (CBD)- from Cannabis

> Cannabinoids refer to any of groups of related compounds that include cannabinol and the active constituents of cannabis. They activate cannabinoid receptors in the body. The body itself produces compounds called endocannabinoids and they play a role in many processes within the body that help to create a healthy environment to treat cancer without any psychoactive effects.

> 'Cannabinoids have been proven to reduce cancer cells as they have a great impact on the rebuilding of the immune system. Although not every strain of cannabis has the same effect, more and more patients are seeing success in cancer reduction in a short period of time by using cannabis. Contrary to popular belief, smoking cannabis does not assist a great deal in treating disease within the body as therapeutic levels cannot be reached through smoking. Creating oil from the plant or eating the plant is the best way to go about getting the necessary ingredients, the cannabinoids.

> (http://www.collective-evolution.com/2014/02/18/molecular-biologist-explains-how-thc-completely-kills-cancer-cells/comment-page-4/ ;March 2015).

There are still controversies in regards to accepting this plant as a medicine rather than a harmful substance. This plant could benefit the planet in more ways than one (clothing, paper, fuel, building, etc.). Although cannabis is not something offered in the same regard as chemotherapy, more people are becoming aware of its healing properties, which is why it's so important to continue to spread information like this. Nobody can really deny the tremendous healing power of cannabis, which has been proven in isolated experiments, and hopefully, it will become popular, especially in treating brain problems.

When THC connects to the CB1 or CB2 cannabinoid receptor site on the cancer cell, it causes an increase in ceramide synthesis which induce cell death.

A normal healthy cell does not produce ceramide in the presence of THC, thus is not affected by the cannabinoid.

The cancer cell dies, not because of cytotoxic chemicals, but because of a tiny little shift in the mitochondria. Within most cells there is in the nucleus, numerous mitochondria (hundreds to thousands), and various other organelles in the cytoplasm. The purpose of the mitochondria is to produce energy (ATP) for cell use [as we learned at the beginning of this chapter]. As ceramide starts to accumulate, turning up the Sphingolipid Rheostat, it increases the mitochondrial membrane pore permeability to cytochrome C, a critical protein in energy synthesis. Cytochrome C is pushed out of the mitochondria, killing the source of energy for the cell.

Ceramide also causes genotoxic stress in the cancer cell nucleus generating a protein called p53, whose job it is to disrupt calcium metabolism in the mitochondria. If this weren't enough, ceramide disrupts the cellular lysosome, the cell's digestive system that provides nutrients for all cell functions. Ceramide, and other sphingolipids, actively inhibit pro-survival pathways in the cell leaving no possibility at all of cancer cell survival.

The key to this process is the accumulation of ceramide in the system. This means taking therapeutic amounts of CBD and THC, steadily, over a period of time, keeping metabolic pressure on this cancer cell death pathway.

How did this pathway come to be? Why is it that the body can take a simple plant enzyme and use it for profound healing in many different physiological systems? [Remember that the Mother Nature prepared all the ingredients for us to heal and recover.]

This endocannabinoid system exists in all animal bodies, just waiting for its matched exocannabinoid activator. Our own endocannabinoid system covers all cells and nerves; it is the messenger of information flowing between our immune system and the central nervous system. It is responsible for neuroprotection, and micro-manages the immune system. This is the primary control system that maintains homeostasis, our well being.

Just out of curiosity, how does the work get done at the cellular level, and where does the body make the endocannabinoids? Here we see that endocannabinoids have their origin in nerve cells right at the synapse. When the body is compromised through illness or injury it calls insistently to the endocannabinoid system and directs the immune system to bring healing. If these homeostatic systems are weakened, it should be no surprise that exocannabinoids are therapeutic. It helps the body in the most natural way possible.

It is known that THC and CBD are biomimetic to anandamide, that's why the body can use both interchangeably. Thus, when stress, injury, or illness demand more from endogenous anandamide than can be produced by the body, its mimetic exocannabinoids are activated. If the stress is transitory, then the treatment can be transitory. If the demand is sustained, such as in cancer, then treatment needs to provide sustained pressure of the modulating agent on the homeostatic systems.

Typically CBD gravitates to the densely packed CB2 receptors in the spleen, home to the body's immune system. From there, immune cells seek out and destroy cancer cells. Interestingly, it has been shown that THC and CBD cannabinoids have the ability to kill cancer cells directly without going through immune intermediaries. THC and CBD hijack the lipoxygenase pathway to directly inhibit tumour growth.

(The above information was collected from the article 'How Cannabis Oil Works to Kill Cancer Cells' written by Dennis Hill; it is found on:http://www. cureyourowncancer.org/how-cannabis-oil-works.html).

One of the latest methods of reaping the benefits of cannabis is juicing.

Juicing is a great way to get the best stuff out of plant materials. It makes digestion easy and allows your body to really make the most of what you put into it. So, it stands to reason that many of the benefits associated with smoking, vaporizing, or eating cannabis could be enhanced through juicing.

High-aside, some argue juicing raw cannabis to be the most beneficial, and it does all of this without getting users stoned. Raw cannabis is not psychoactive. The beneficial compounds within are known as cannabidiols (CBD) and they are not the THC responsible for getting you high.

(http://themindunleashed.org/2014/03/woman-
replaces-40-medications-raw-cannabis-juice.html-
March 2015)

The problem is that in many countries, including Australia, you cannot buy cannabis or you are not allowed to grow it in your backyard because of its psychoactive effect (or so they say). My question is, why there is no medicinal cannabis without the psychedelic effect found in the health shops when everybody knows how therapeutic it is? Maybe it's because somebody wants people to stay sick and buy expensive pills to fill the corporations' pockets! That's why it is illegal; it doesn't make money for them!

This healing plant should be available for everybody to grow and use it to heal without spending so much money on expensive medicine and treatments; because God gave it to us for free.

While some critics say you would have to juice quite an extensive amount of cannabis to get enough of its benefits, this could become more feasible as marijuana continues to be deregulated.

Nature has designed the perfect medicine in plants that fits exactly with our own immune system to provide rapid and complete immune response for systemic integrity and cure for any disease; we just need to acknowledge and use them.

See more at the following:

http://cannabisnationradio.com/dennis-hill-cytotoxicity

US National Library of Medicine National Institutes of Health—Pub Med

http://www.hempforfuture.com/2014/03/26/molecular-biologist-explains-how-thc-completely-kills-cancer/

http://www.youtube.com/watch?v=G_5SpCgfi10#t=68

http://www.youtube.com/watch?v=JWklpCxg2jc

www.cureyourowncancer.org/scientific-studies

http://themindunleashed.org/2014/03/woman-replaces-40-medications-raw-cannabis-juice.html

http://youtu.be/75FQKQOKvVM

http://www.cureyourowncancer.org/how-cannabis-oil-works.html.

And to accompany those powerful cancer killers mentioned above, we have some powerful vegetables, fruits, and herbs which will also contribute to free our body from cancer.

What diet we should have when fighting cancer?

'You are what you eat.' You've heard this expression many times, and it is true. All the food and drinks which we put in our mouth are stored in the body and filtrated through the liver and kidney. All these substances are used to build our muscles, bones, and organs, and it's up to us to choose whether to create our body from clean organic materials or from chemicals and hormones derived from the plants and animals we eat.

We cannot talk about building and healing our body without talking about the liver.

The liver is the body's second largest organ, weighing in at around 3 pounds, and it is the cleanser and filter of the bloodstream. The liver performs many essential functions—digestion, metabolism, immunity, and the storage of nutrients within the body. These functions make the liver a vital organ, and without it, the tissues of the body would quickly die from lack of energy and nutrients.

Let's have a quick look at the bodily functions performed by the liver.

(The following information/classification was collected from the website: http://www.innerbody.com/image_digeov/card10-new2. html#full-description ;March 2015)

1. Digestion

The liver plays an active role in the process of digestion through the production of *bile*. Bile is a mixture of the bilirubin pigment, water, bile salts, and cholesterol. The fatty acids in the blood passing through the liver are absorbed by hepatocytes (the liver cells) and are metabolized to produce energy in the form of ATP.

> Glycerol, another lipid component, is converted into glucose by hepatocytes through the process of gluconeogenesis. Hepatocytes can also produce lipids like cholesterol, phospholipids, and lipoproteins that are used by other cells throughout the body. Much of the cholesterol produced by hepatocytes gets excreted from the body as a component of bile.

Our **digestive system** breaks down carbohydrates into the monosaccharide glucose, which cells use as a primary energy source. Blood entering the liver through the hepatic portal vein is extremely rich in glucose from digested food. Hepatocytes absorb much of this glucose and store it as the macromolecule glycogen, a branched polysaccharide that allows the hepatocytes to pack away large amounts of glucose and quickly release glucose between meals. The absorption and release of glucose by the hepatocytes helps to maintain homeostasis and protects the rest of the body from dangerous spikes and drops in the blood glucose level.

2. Detoxification

As blood from the digestive organs passes through the hepatic portal circulation, the hepatocytes of the liver monitor the contents of the blood and remove many potentially toxic substances before they can reach the rest of the body. Enzymes in hepatocytes metabolize many of these toxins such as alcohol and drugs into their inactive metabolites. And in order to keep hormone levels within homeostatic limits, the liver also metabolizes and removes from circulation hormones produced by the body's own glands.

The detoxification function of the liver is the most important issue you need to keep in mind when dealing with cancer. If the liver is sick and can't eliminate the excessive toxins produced by the cancer, those will accumulate in the body and poison it, compromising your health results.

3. Storage

'The liver provides storage of many essential nutrients, vitamins, and minerals obtained from blood passing through the hepatic portal system. Glucose is transported into hepatocytes under the influence of the hormone insulin and stored as the polysaccharide glycogen. Hepatocytes also absorb and store fatty acids from digested triglycerides. The storage of these nutrients allows the liver to maintain the homeostasis of blood glucose. Our liver also stores **vitamins and minerals**—such as vitamins A, D, E, K, and B12, and the minerals iron and copper—in order to provide a constant supply of these essential substances to the tissues of the body.

4. Production

The liver is responsible for the production of several vital protein components of blood plasma: prothrombin, fibrinogen, and albumins. Prothrombin and fibrinogen proteins are coagulation factors involved in the formation of blood clots. Albumins are proteins that maintain the isotonic environment of the blood so that cells of the body do not gain or lose water in the presence of body fluids.

5. Immunity

The liver functions as an organ of the **immune system** through the function of the Kupffer cells that line the sinusoids. Kupffer cells are a type of fixed macrophage that form part of the mononuclear phagocyte system along with macrophages in the spleen and **lymph nodes**. Kupffer cells play an important role by capturing and digesting bacteria, fungi, parasites, worn-out blood cells, and cellular debris. The large volume of blood passing through the hepatic portal system and the liver allows Kupffer cells to clean large volumes of blood very quickly.'

In this century, our liver needs to do a high amount of work to keep our body clean, as thousands of chemicals are added to food and over 700 have been identified in drinking water. Plants are sprayed with toxic chemicals, animals are injected with potent hormones, and antibiotics and a significant amount of our food are genetically engineered, processed, refined, frozen, and cooked.

All this can lead to destruction of delicate vitamins and minerals, which are needed for the detoxification pathways in the liver. The liver must try to cope with every toxic chemical in our environment, as well as damaged fats that are present in processed and fried foods. [So stop eating fast food!]

They are hormonally active substances which means they can cross placental barriers and may have profound effects on the offspring of animals which ingest them. The types of chemicals that mimic hormones are as diverse as pesticides, herbicides, fertilizers, plastics, solvents, and more.

> Richard M. Sharpe, research physiologist with the Medical Research Council in Edinburgh, hypothesized that oestrogens in the environment can disrupt the body's hormonal balance, possibly explaining phenomena such as earlier puberty, lowered sperm counts, and other reproductive anomalies exhibited by late 20th century females and males of many species. Sharp says: 'Of all the hormones we know, the oestrogens are the most

potent. You can get biological effects from oestrogen at levels so low you cannot measure them by any analytical method'. Other environmentalists and scientists postulate effects ranging from behavioural changes to motor, intellectual, reproductive and immune system impairment.

Ingestion or exposure to these substances can have dramatic effects on our state of health and the development of disease [especially of cancer].

In oestrogen sensitive breast tumours it is important to regulate oestrogen metabolites. There are 2 pathways which oestrogen may be metabolized to estrone. Altering the ratio of these two pathways has a dramatic effect on the long term survival of the patient.'(http://www.innerbody.com/image_digeov/card10-new2.html ;March 2015).

'As many other human pathologic conditions, end-stage liver disease goes hand in hand with oxidative stress, which refers to damage inflicted to biological tissues by reactive oxygen molecules. Such molecules, also called free radicals, occur naturally as a byproduct of metabolic processes in the body and are associated with many chronic diseases including cancer, diabetes, neurodegenerative and cardiovascular diseases.'(http://medicalxpress.com/news/2014-04-scientists-critical-end-stage-liver-discovery.html- March 2015).

'The liver filter is designed to remove toxic matter such as dead cells, microorganisms, chemicals, drugs and particulate debris from the bloodstream. The liver filter is called the sinusoidal system, and contains specialized cells known as Kupffer cells which ingest and break down toxic matter.'(https://www.liverdoctor.com/liver/the-liver-and-detoxification/; March 2015).

That's why, in our battle with cancer, we need to accord great importance to cleansing the liver, as it is overloaded with residual products from the cancer's activity or from our meals composed of poisonous meat (processed meat or meat from animals treated with hormones) or vegetables (grown with chemicals and treated with pesticides).

Read more about the liver's function at http://medicalxpress.com/news/2014-04-scientists-critical-end-stage-liver-discovery.html.

'A liver cleanse is a natural procedure designed to detoxify, flush, and purge the liver of fatty deposits, built up toxins, and accumulated stones. Most liver cleanse programs also include a gallbladder cleanse which helps purge the gallbladder of gallstones. Liver stones are formed when excess cholesterol crystallizes into small pebble size stones.'(http://www.globalhealingcenter.com/liver-cleanse-kit.html ; March 2015).

Usually, a liver cleanse involves eating a healthy organic diet and drinking an organic herbal liver-cleansing mixture associated with enemas to stimulate and detoxify the liver.

There are a few ways to clean the liver.

1.   Coffee Enemas and Warm Compresses

A coffee enema is the enema-related procedure of inserting coffee into the anus to cleanse the rectum and the large intestines.

> The first mention of the enema in medical literature is in the Ancient Egyptian Ebers Papyrus (c 1550 BCE). Many medications were administered by enemas. There was a Keeper of the Royal Rectum who may have primarily been the pharaoh's enema maker.
>
> The Olmec from their middle preclassic period (10th through 7th centuries BCE) through the Spanish Conquest used trance-inducing substances ceremonially, and these were ingested by, among other routes, via enemas administered using jars.

The Maya in their late classic age (7th through 10th centuries CE) used enemas for, at least, ritual purposes, in the Xibalban court of the God D whose worship included ritual cult paraphernalia.

In the 2nd century CE the Greek philosopher Celsus recommended an enema of pearl barley in milk or rose oil with butter as a nutrient for those suffering from dysentery and unable to eat and Galen mentions enemas in several contexts. (https://en.wikipedia.org/wiki/Enema, April 2015)

In early 1900s, coffee enema was mentioned as a stimulant and as a treatment for shock in medical and nursing textbooks, and it was considered to have an anticancer effect by 'detoxifying' the metabolic products of tumours and other toxins held in our bodies. Also, it was considered to have other benefits like cleaning the liver, healing bowel diseases, eliminating parasites, helping with depression and general nervous tension, decreasing blood pressure, and eliminating pain.

In 1958, Dr Max Gerson collected a series of results from his patients treated with raw juices and coffee enema for his book "*A Cancer Therapy: Results of Fifty Cases*", as a proof of the coffee enema's efficacy.

Gerson's therapy included up to six enemas per day (one at every four hours), which in my opinion will wash out the entire protective layer of mucus of the colon—and good bacteria.

It is wise to be balanced in everything we do. Do not exaggerate, and always ask your body what it needs.

Dr Gerson's method is used today at several clinics, most of which are in Mexico and Europe.

The enema mechanically washes out the colon, removing toxic substances and often nests of parasites, bacteria, yeast colonies, and other debris.

Repeated enemas also stimulate the colon slightly by dilating it and improve food absorption by cleaning out all the old food deposits and impacted faeces from the bowel pockets (diverticulum). These are slight expansions or dilations in the wall of the colon which trap food particles, bacteria, and often harbour parasitic organisms, such as worms and yeasts.

Another mechanical effect is to increase peristalsis (the movement); it causes the colon to become active, emptying its contents more completely. Certain food items, especially refined white flour, can turn hard in the colon and stick to its walls.

In cancer, coffee enema is recommended to detoxify the body and eliminate the toxins and chemicals from the tumour activity.

Most coffees contain very useful substances like antioxidants; selenium; acids such as caffeic, ferulic, and chlorogenic acid; salts of palmitic acid, which enhance glutathione S-transferase (an important enzyme in the liver); and other acids and minerals.

To do a coffee enema, you need to use a colonic irrigation machine, an enema bucket or bag, or even a rubber pump, like the one used in vaginal wash (but this method is harder and messy as you need to refill the pump two to three times).

One of the most common procedure to prepare coffee enemas is to boil 1–2 tablespoons of organic coffee in a cup of water. When the coffee reaches the boiling point, stop the burner and let the coffee steam (covered) for five to ten minutes. Add another cup of cold water—or less—until it's the right temperature for your body, then strain it. The obtained solution can be used for enemas and needs to be retained for fifteen to thirty minutes while you relax on your side or lie on your back. Start with a short time and a small quantity, and increase gradually.

A trick for the beginners, if you can't hold it for fifteen minutes, is to first have a small enema for a short time to clean the colon, than the real fifteen-minute enema. Having bowel movement before doing your enema will help in holding the coffee for a longer time.

At the beginning, it will be difficult to retain the coffee, but with patience, you will manage to do it after a while. I know a naturopath who does it two to three times per day; I personally wasn't able to do enemas to treat my cancer.

Read more about enemas at http://www.treating-cancer-alternatively. com/Coffee-enemas.html#basis or at http://www.raw-wisdom.com/ coffee-enemas.

A real help in cleansing the liver are also the warm compresses applied over the liver. There are a few plants used as essential oils, referred to as hepatic, which have a tonic and beneficial action on the liver and strengthen its various actions.

> By the far the most important of these is Rosemary, which stimulates the production and flow of bile, helps in cases of jaundice and is a general liver tonic. Other helpful oils are Camomile and Peppermint, which benefit the liver and the digestive system as a whole, Cypress, Lemon and Thyme which are useful when the liver is congested, and Juniper as an aid to detoxification.

> General body massage or baths with these oils will enable them to enter the bloodstream and reach the liver quite quickly, but relief from discomfort in the liver area is best achieved by means of warm (not too hot) compresses over the liver. In cases of jaundice and congestion, alternating hot and cold compresses, finishing with a cold one, will stimulate the liver and improve its circulation and function. (http://www. oilsandplants.com/liver.htm- March 2015)

Be aware that not all oils are good and that some essential oils which are described as toxic are all nearly capable of damaging the liver to the extent where very serious illness or even death could follow.

You can also use castor oil, which is derived from the castor bean (*Ricinus communis*).

A castor oil pack made by soaking a piece of flannel in castor oil (the flannel is covered with a sheet of plastic, and then a hot water bottle is placed over the plastic to heat the pack) is placed on the skin to increase circulation and to promote elimination and healing of the tissues and organs underneath the skin. It is used to stimulate the liver, relieve pain, increase lymphatic circulation, reduce inflammation, and improve digestion.

If you don't have those oils, you can do a very concentrated tea of the plants described above or other hepatic plants, such as Great Celandine (*Chelidonium Majus*), St John's wort (*Hypericum Perforatum*), Garden Marigold (*Calendula Officinalis*), St Mary's Thistle (*Sylibum Marianum*), Yarrow (*Achillea millefolium*), etc.

Dip the compress cloths into the tea, wring it out, and apply it on the liver region, then cover it with a warm towel and apply a warm heat bag/water bottle on top. Lie down for more than thirty minutes, relax, and keep warm.

2. Herbal Tea

Another detoxification method is drinking herbal tea. What types of tea can we use to help the liver?

> We hear about it all the time; tea is loaded with anti-oxidants and cancer fighting benefits.
>
> There are some trustworthy companies that provide quality organic teas to its consumers by monitoring the amount of pesticides and also using sustainable farming methods and fair trade standards. Some of these include: Teatulia, Numi, Zhyna's Gypsy Tea, Choice Organics, Traditional Medicinals, Rishi and many more; you just have to search. Even though brands like this are a little

more expensive than the conventional ones, it is well worth it. Not only will you be getting the full benefit that the tea has to offer, you will be supporting ethical, sustainable and organic farming practices. The more people that switch to brands like these, the greater push conventional brands will feel to start changing their practices and principles [and become organic].

Tea can definitely be a great way to boost your health. Black, green, white, oolong and pu-erh teas all come from the Camellia Sinensis plant that is native to China and India. These teas contain many anti-oxidants called flavonoids; the most potent of these are known as ECGC and can help against free radicals that can contribute to a variety of cancers and heart disease. Many herbal teas contain some pretty amazing health benefits [and they have been used for millennia].' (http://www.collective-evolution.com/2013/10/26/whats-in-your-mug-the-toxic-truth-about-tea/ ; March 2015)

The most common teas used in liver detoxification are the following:

a.   Greater Celandine (*Chelidonium majus*)

Celandine tea has multiple actions and can be used both internally and externally. Internally, it stimulates and regulates the secretion of bile, stimulates gall bladder tone (improves bile flow). It is an important hepatoprotective, helps in the normalization of bilirubin and cholesterol, and helps in renal lithiasis. It is analgesic, antispasmodic, anti-inflammatory, antibacterial, antiviral, and antitumor. Last but not least, it serves as a sedative and narcotic on the central nervous system.

Internally, it is used as an adjuvant in biliary dyskinesia, acute and chronic cholecystitis, biliary colic, chronic hepatitis, liver cirrhosis, gallstones, gastrointestinal tract spasms, spastic cough, and tumours in the oesophagus, pancreas, liver, or lungs.

For internal action, celandine tea is prepared as follows: put half a teaspoon of celandine to 250 millilitres of hot water, then leave it to infuse for ten minutes before being consumed. The treatment period is ten days, then take a break for a few weeks and start again.

Externally, it is used as an antibacterial and antifungal adjuvant in wounds, fistulas, dermatitis, psoriasis, chronic skin infections, warts, corns, keratitis, and skin tumours. If being used for skin problems, prepare the ointment: 40 grams powdered celandine, 20 grams lanolin, and 20 grams petroleum jelly.

b.   St John's wort (*Hypericum perforatum*)

St John's wort has antiseptic, anti-inflammatory, decongestant, disinfectant, astringent, antidiarrhoeal healing effects due to the presence of chlorogenic acid, hypericin, and pseudohypericin. Also, it has cholagogue action (promotes the discharge of bile), is a stimulant of digestion, decreases stomach acid, is hypotensive, helps remove excess water from the body. Due to volatile oils, it also has a calming and sedative effect on the nervous system.

St John's wort is recommended in digestive disorders (gastritis, hyperacidity, peptic ulcer gastro, enterocolitis, biliary dyskinesia, hepatitis), fluid retention (edema, ascites), hypertension, autonomic dystonia, psychomotor agitation, panic attacks, depression, irritability, insomnia, nervous disorders in menopause, and in liver cleansing and support.

For its administration, the infusion is prepared from a teaspoon of chopped herb in a cup of boiling water; it is left to brew for fifteen to twenty minutes, then strained. Drink two to three cups a day.

As for precautions and contraindications, treatment with St John's wort is better not to last more than two months. After a month- long, it can be resumed to avoid unwanted symptoms in neuralgia, headache, photosensitivity (the phenomenon of sensitization to light) and can be continued after a short break.

c. <u>St Mary's thistle (*Sylibum marianum*)</u>

St Mary's thistle can be considered as the liver's police officer.

> 'St Mary's Thistle, or Milk Thistle, is named after the herb's most active constituent and is one of the most protective liver herbs. The part of the plant containing most of these constituents is the fruit of the thistle. It has antioxidant, liver protective and restorative properties as well as the ability to assist bile production. It is often used to aid the digestion of fat in the small intestine and bile is necessary for us to be able to excrete substances our body no longer needs such as old sex hormones. Without enough bile, these hormones can get recycled which can lead to poor energy and weight gain, amongst other things.
>
> With more research in modern western herbal medicine our understanding of Milk Thistle's clinical use has widened to include treatment of jaundice, gall stones, colic, hepatitis, reducing cholesterol, stabilizing blood glucose levels, non-alcoholic fatty liver disease (often caused by an intolerance or an over consumption of grains or fructose) and liver damage from alcohol and drugs. Milk thistle has been clinically proven to lower specific liver enzymes often tested in standard blood tests that indicate liver damage.
>
> Silymarin, an extract from the seed, acts on the membranes of the liver cells preventing the entry of virus toxins and other toxic compounds and improving liver regeneration in hepatitis, cirrhosis, mushroom poisoning and other diseases of the liver. All parts of the plant are used as infusions, tinctures, or as an extract with the strongest concentration being in the seeds.

To make tea from the leaves, which are highly effective as well, use 1 tsp dried, fine cut leaves or 3 full tsp fresh leaves. Pour boiling water, let it to stay for 10 mins and drink 3 times a day'.

(http://happyherbcompany.com/saintmarysthistle December 2014)

'The load we place on our liver through modern day life is highly underestimated as we are frequently exposed to a plethora of chemicals in our environment, food, cosmetics, medications, agricultural sprays and preservatives. Not to mention the development of chronic disease such as diabetes, cardiovascular disease, cancer, cholesterol and obesity. Milk Thistle is the herb of choice for many of these conditions and diseases and is clinically safe to use in conjunction with many medications prescribed today.' (https://www.drlibby.com/blogs/St_Mary_s_Thistle___The_Liver_s_Protector ; March 2015)

3. Vegetables and Fruits

There are many foods that can help cleanse the liver naturally by stimulating its natural ability to clean toxic waste from the body.

1. Garlic

'Just a small amount of this pungent white bulb has the ability to activate liver enzymes that help your body flush out toxins. Garlic also holds high amounts of allicin and selenium, two natural compounds that aid in liver cleansing.

2. Grapefruit

High in both vitamin C and antioxidants, grapefruit increases the natural cleansing processes of the liver. A small glass of freshly-squeezed grapefruit juice will help boost production of the liver detoxification enzymes that help flush out carcinogens and other toxins.

3. Beets and Carrots

Both are extremely high in plant-flavonoids and beta-carotene; eating beets and carrots can help stimulate and improve overall liver function.

4. Green Tea

This liver-loving beverage is full of plant antioxidants known as catechins, a compound known to assist liver function. Green tea is not only delicious, it's also a great way to improve your overall diet.

5. Leafy Green Vegetables

One of our most powerful allay in cleansing the liver, leafy greens can be eaten raw, cooked, or juiced. Extremely high in plant chlorophylls, greens suck up environmental toxins from the blood stream. With their distinct ability to <u>neutralize heavy metals</u>, chemicals and pesticides, these cleansing foods offer a powerful protective mechanism for the liver. Make sure they are organic and not loaded with pesticides.

Try incorporating leafy greens such as bitter gourd, arugula, dandelion greens, spinach, mustard greens, and chicory into your diet. This will help increase the creation and flow of bile, the substance that removes waste from the organs and blood.

6. Avocados

This nutrient-dense super-food helps the body produce glutathione, a compound that is necessary for the liver to cleanse harmful toxins.

7. Apples

High in pectin, apples hold the chemical constituents necessary for the body to cleanse and release toxins from the digestive tract. This, in turn, makes it easier for the liver to handle the toxic load during the cleansing process.

8. Olive Oil

Cold-pressed organic oils such as olive, hemp and flax-seed are great for the liver, when used in moderation. They help the body by providing a lipid base which can collect harmful toxins from the body. In this way, it takes some of the burden off the liver in terms of the toxic overload many of us suffer from.

9. Alternative Grains

It's not only that you need alternative grains like quinoa, millet, and buckwheat in your diet, it's that if you've got wheat, flour, or other whole grains in your diet, it's time to make changes. Your liver is your body's filter for toxins, and grains that contain gluten are full of them. A study last year found that persons who experienced gluten sensitivities also had abnormal liver enzyme test results, and that's just one of many.

10. Cruciferous Vegetables

Eating broccoli and cauliflower will increase the amount of glucosinolate in your system, adding to enzyme production in the liver. These natural enzymes help flush out carcinogens, and other toxins, out of our body which may significantly lower risks associated with cancer.

Much like broccoli and cauliflower, eating cabbage helps stimulate the activation of two crucial liver detoxifying enzymes that help flush out toxins. Try eating more kimchi, coleslaw, cabbage soup and sauerkraut

11. Lemons & Limes

These citrus fruits contain very high amounts of vitamin C, which aids the body in synthesizing toxic materials into substances that can be absorbed by water. Drinking freshly-squeezed lemon or lime juice in the morning helps stimulate the liver and also alkalinising the blood.

12. Walnuts

Holding high amounts of the amino acid arginine, walnuts aid the liver in detoxifying ammonia. Walnuts are also high in glutathione and omega-3 fatty acids, which support normal liver cleansing actions. Make sure you chew the nuts well (until they are liquefied) before swallowing, for a better result.

13. Turmeric

The liver's favourite spice. Try adding some of this detoxifying goodness into your next lentil stew or veggie dish for an instant liver pick-me-up. Turmeric helps boost liver detox, by assisting enzymes that actively flush out dietary carcinogens [we talked about it already].

Other liver cleanse foods not listed above include artichoke, asparagus, kale, and brussel sprouts. Eating fresh foods is a great way to help keep your liver functioning properly and the best way to do it is juicing or blending the vegetables and fruits'. (http://www.globalhealingcenter.com/natural-health/liver-cleanse-foods/ ; March 2015)

It is very important that you start slow on juicing, as it could make you feel sick at first. Drink a small amount at first (such as 1/4 cup), and slowly build up to higher amounts. The beet juice will cause your liver to dump toxins into your system, as it is a very good liver cleanser.

Talking about juicing will take us to the wide range of vegetable and fruits which we can eat. You need to know that there are some specific vegetables recommended for cancer treatment, and we will discuss them here. Before anything else, we need to understand the meaning of acidic and basic food.

Human blood pH should be slightly alkaline (7.35–7.45). Below or above this range means symptoms and disease. A pH of 7.0 is neutral. A pH below 7.0 is acidic. A pH above 7.0 is alkaline.

An acidic pH can occur from, an acid forming diet, emotional stress, toxic overload, and/or immune reactions or any process that deprives the cells of oxygen and other nutrients. The body will try to compensate for acidic pH by using alkaline minerals. If the diet does not contain enough minerals to compensate, a build up of acids in the cells will occur.

An acidic balance will: decrease the body's ability to absorb minerals and other nutrients, decrease the energy production in the cells, decrease its ability to repair damaged cells, decrease its ability to detoxify heavy metals, make tumour cells thrive, and make it more susceptible to fatigue and illness. A blood pH less than 6.8, (which is only slightly acidic), can induce coma and death.

The reason acidosis is more common in our society is mostly due to the typical American diet, which is far too high in acid producing animal products like meat, eggs and dairy, and far too low in alkaline producing foods like fresh vegetables. Additionally, we eat acid producing processed foods like white flour and sugar and drink acid producing beverages like coffee and soft drinks. We use too many drugs, which are acid forming; and we use artificial chemical sweeteners like NutraSweet, Spoonful, Sweet 'N Low, Equal, or Aspartame, which are poison and extremely acid forming. One of the best things we can do to correct an overly acid body is to change the diet and lifestyle.

To maintain health, the diet should consist of 60% alkaline forming foods and 40% acid forming foods. To restore health, the diet should consist of 80% alkaline forming foods and 20% acid forming foods.

Generally, alkaline forming foods include: most fruits, green vegetables, peas, beans, lentils, spices, herbs and seasonings, and seeds and nuts.

Generally, acid forming foods include: meat, fish, poultry, eggs, grains, and legumes.

This chart is for those trying to 'adjust' their body pH The pH scale is from 0 to 14, with numbers below 7 acidic (low on oxygen) and numbers above 7 alkaline. An acidic body is a sickness magnet. What you eat and drink will impact where your body's pH level falls.

Balance is the Key!!!

This chart is intended only as a general guide to alkalizing and acidifying foods.'(www.rense.com/1. mpicons/acidalka.htm; December 2014).

...ALKALINE FOODS...	...ACIDIC FOODS...
ALKALIZING VEGETABLES	**ACIDIFYING VEGETABLES**
Alfalfa	Corn
Barley Grass	Lentils
Beet Greens	Olives
Beets	Winter Squash
Broccoli	
Cabbage	**ACIDIFYING FRUITS**
Carrot	Blueberries
Cauliflower	Canned or Glazed Fruits
Celery	Cranberries
Chard Greens	Currants
Chlorella	Plums**
Collard Greens	Prunes**
Cucumber	
Dandelions	**ACIDIFYING GRAINS,**
Dulce	**GRAIN PRODUCTS**
Edible Flowers	Amaranth
Eggplant	Barley
Fermented Veggies	Bran, oat
Garlic	Bran, wheat
Green Beans	Bread
Green Peas	Corn
Kale	Cornstarch
Kohlrabi	Crackers, soda
Lettuce	Flour, wheat
Mushrooms	Flour, white
Mustard Greens	Hemp Seed Flour
Nightshade Veggies	Kamut
Onions	Macaroni
Parsnips (high glycemic)	Noodles
Peas	Oatmeal
Peppers	Oats (rolled)
Pumpkin	Quinoa
Radishes	Rice (all)
Rutabaga	Rice Cakes

Sea Veggies
Spinach, green
Spirulina
Sprouts
Sweet Potatoes
Tomatoes
Watercress
Wheat Grass
Wild Greens

ALKALIZING ORIENTAL VEGETABLES

Daikon
Dandelion Root
Kombu
Maitake
Nori
Reishi
Shitake
Umeboshi
Wakame

ALKALIZING FRUITS

Apple
Apricot
Avocado
Banana (high glycemic)
Berries
Blackberries
Cantaloupe
Cherries, sour
Coconut, fresh
Currants
Dates, dried
Figs, dried
Grapes
Grapefruit

Rye
Spaghetti
Spelt
Wheat Germ
Wheat

ACIDIFYING BEANS & LEGUMES

Almond Milk
Black Beans
Chick Peas
Green Peas
Kidney Beans
Lentils
Pinto Beans
Red Beans
Rice Milk
Soy Beans
Soy Milk
White Beans

ACIDIFYING DAIRY

Butter
Cheese
Cheese, Processed
Ice Cream
Ice Milk

ACIDIFYING NUTS & BUTTERS

Cashews
Legumes
Peanut Butter
Peanuts
Pecans
Tahini
Walnuts

Honeydew Melon
Lemon
Lime
Muskmelons
Nectarine
Orange
Peach
Pear
Pineapple
Raisins
Raspberries
Rhubarb
Strawberries
Tangerine
Tomato
Tropical Fruits
Umeboshi Plums
Watermelon

ALKALIZING PROTEIN
Almonds
Chestnuts
Millet
Tempeh (fermented)
Tofu (fermented)
Whey Protein Powder

ALKALIZING SWEETENERS
Stevia

**ALKALIZING SPICES &
SEASONINGS**
Chili Pepper
Cinnamon
Curry
Ginger
Herbs (all)

**ACIDIFYING ANIMAL
PROTEIN**
Bacon
Beef
Carp
Clams
Cod
Corned Beef
Fish
Haddock
Lamb
Lobster
Mussels
Organ Meats
Oyster
Pike
Pork
Rabbit
Salmon
Sardines
Sausage
Scallops
Shellfish
Shrimp
Tuna
Turkey
Veal
Venison

ACIDIFYING FATS & OILS
Avacado Oil
Butter
Canola Oil
Corn Oil
Flax Oil
Hemp Seed Oil
Lard

Miso
Mustard
Sea Salt
Tamari

ALKALIZING OTHER
Alkaline Antioxidant Water
Apple Cider Vinegar
Bee Pollen
Fresh Fruit Juice
Green Juices
Lecithin Granules
Mineral Water
Molasses, blackstrap
Probiotic Cultures
Soured Dairy Products
Veggie Juices

ALKALIZING MINERALS
Calcium: pH 12
Cesium: pH 14
Magnesium: pH 9
Potassium: pH 14
Sodium: pH 14

Although it might seem that citrus fruits would have an acidifying effect on the body, the citric acid they contain actually has an alkalinizing effect in the system.

Olive Oil
Safflower Oil
Sesame Oil
Sunflower Oil

ACIDIFYING SWEETENERS
Carob
Corn Syrup
Sugar

ACIDIFYING ALCOHOL
Beer
Hard Liquor
Spirits
Wine

ACIDIFYING OTHER FOODS
Catsup
Cocoa
Coffee
Mustard
Pepper
Soft Drinks
Vinegar

ACIDIFYING DRUGS & CHEMICALS
Aspirin
Chemicals
Drugs, Medicinal
Drugs, Psychedelic
Herbicides
Pesticides
Tobacco

Note that a food's acid or alkaline forming tendency in the body has nothing to do with the actual pH of the food itself. For example, lemons are very acidic, however the end products they produce after digestion and assimilation are very alkaline so, lemons are alkaline forming in the body. Likewise, meat will test alkaline before digestion, but it leaves very acidic residue in the body so, like nearly all animal products, meat is very acid forming.

ACIDIFYING JUNK FOOD
Beer: pH 2.5
Coca-Cola: pH 2
Coffee: pH 4

Extremely Alkaline
Lemons, watermelon.

Alkaline Forming
Cantaloupe, cayenne celery, dates, figs, kelp, limes, mango, melons, papaya, parsley, seaweeds, seedless grapes (sweet), watercress.
Asparagus, fruit juices, grapes (sweet), kiwifruit, passionfruit, pears (sweet), pineapple, raisins, umeboshi plums, and vegetable juices.

Moderately Alkaline
Apples (sweet), alfalfa sprouts, apricots, avocados, bananas (ripe), currants, dates, figs (fresh), garlic, grapefruit, grapes (less sweet), guavas, herbs (leafy green), lettuce (leafy green), nectarine, peaches (sweet), pears (less sweet), peas (fresh, sweet), pumpkin (sweet), sea salt (vegetable).
Apples (sour), beans (fresh, green), beets, bell peppers, broccoli, cabbage, carob, cauliflower, ginger (fresh), grapes (sour), lettuce (pale green), oranges, peaches (less sweet), peas (less sweet), potatoes (with skin), pumpkin (less sweet), raspberries, strawberries, squash, sweet Corn (fresh), turnip, vinegar (apple cider).

Slightly Alkaline

Almonds, artichokes (jerusalem), brussel sprouts, cherries, coconut (fresh), cucumbers, eggplant, honey (raw), leeks, mushrooms, okra, olives (ripe), onions, pickles (homemade), radishes, sea salt, spices, tomatoes (sweet), vinegar (sweet brown rice).

Chestnuts (dry, roasted), egg yolks (soft cooked), essene bread, goat's milk and whey (raw), mayonnaise (homemade), olive oil, sesame seeds (whole), soy beans (dry), soy cheese, soy milk, sprouted grains, tofu, tomatoes (less sweet), and yeast (nutritional flakes).

Neutral

Butter (fresh, unsalted), cream (fresh, raw), cow's milk and whey (raw), margine, oils (except olive), and yogurt (plain).

Moderately Acidic

Bananas (green), barley (rye), blueberries, bran, butter, cereals (unrefined), cheeses, crackers (unrefined rye, rice and wheat), cranberries, dried beans (mung, adzuki, pinto, kidney, garbanzo), dry coconut, egg whites, eggs whole (cooked hard), fructose, goat's milk (homogenized), honey (pasteurized), ketchup, maple syrup (unprocessed), milk (homogenized).

Molasses (unsulferd and organic), most nuts, mustard, oats (rye, organic), olives (pickled), pasta (whole grain), pastry (whole grain and honey), plums, popcorn (with salt and/or butter), potatoes, prunes, rice (basmati and brown), seeds (pumpkin, sunflower), soy sauce, and wheat bread (sprouted organic).

Extremely Acidic

Artificial sweeteners, beef, beer, breads, brown sugar, carbonated soft drinks, cereals (refined), chocolate, cigarettes and tobacco, coffee, cream of wheat (unrefined), custard (with white sugar), deer, drugs, fish, flour (white, wheat), fruit juices with sugar, jams, jellies, lamb.

Liquor, maple syrup (processed), molasses (sulphured), pasta (white), pastries and cakes from white flour, pickles (commercial), pork, poultry, seafood, sugar (white), table salt (refined and iodized), tea (black), white bread, white vinegar (processed), whole wheat foods, wine, and yogurt (sweetened).

See these charts at the following:

http://www.rense.com/1.mpicons/acidalka.htm

http://www.essense-of-life.com/.

A number of studies in the past have shown interesting in vivo results surrounding the use of sodium bicarbonate on cancer tumours. While research is not fully complete on the matter, early results are already showing some powerful effects of tumour metastasis. This of course encourages funding for further research.

Dr. Robert J. Gillies and his colleagues have already demonstrated the effectiveness of baking soda in alkalinizing the area around tumours in mice. The same researchers found that bicarbonate increases tumour pH and also inhibits spontaneous metastases in mice with breast cancer. [If we combine baking soda with lemons, which are the most alkaline fruit, we obtain the best alkalinizing solution.]

Lemon has shown to contain anti-carcinogenic properties as it contains limonoides which are phytochemicals found in a number of citrus fruits. Lemon also has been shown to have strong anti-microbial effects [helping to clean the body of them].

Lemons are also effective in helping the body detoxify. They are rich in vitamin C and help your body neutralize cell-damaging free radicals. Limonene, a substance found in lemons also helps to stimulate lymph flow which is important in removing carcinogens from the body. A weak or under performing lymph system is a big part of disease promotion.

Lemon is also used to help balance Ph. They are taken together with baking soda as it is believed that lemon is one of the safest ways to introduce high alkaline substances into the system. These methods of treatment are able to approach carcinogenic cells and destroy them without destroying healthy cells [as the chemotherapy is doing].

Together lemon and baking soda help to fight cancerous cells or diseases in the body while helping to increase the body's ability to clean itself up of what may be causing the diseases in the first place. Having lemon as a part of your diet is certainly healthy and taking this combination as a detox can also be helpful even if you don't have an illness.

One method I have found for introducing this into your body as a drink is to mix 1/2 a teaspoon of baking soda into 250ml of water with about 1 half of a lemon juice [or more if you like]. Please check into more recipes that might work for you.(http://www.collective-evolution.com/2014/04/15/lemon-baking-soda-shown-to-be-powerful-healing-combination/;December/2014).

We cannot talk about the best types of food without talking about fasting. Some researches show that fasting is an important way to help the body fight cancer.

A recent study has found that "a three-day long fast can regenerate your entire immune system, even if you're elderly. The researchers described the findings as 'remarkable'. Fasting for a few days, they found, has the power to kick-start your stem cells into producing more white blood cells, which are part of your body's natural defence arsenal. As reported by Daily Life:

'Scientists at the University of Southern California (USC) say the discovery could be particularly beneficial for those

suffering from damaged immune systems, such as cancer patients on chemotherapy. It could also help the elderly whose immune systems become less effective . . .

'And the good news is that the body got rid of the parts of the system that might be damaged or old, the inefficient parts, during the fasting. Now, if you start with a system heavily damaged by chemotherapy or ageing, fasting cycles can generate, literally, a new immune system.'

They discovered that longer fasts (two to four days) led to the reduction of an enzyme called protein kinase A (PKA), which previous research has linked to life extension in simple organisms. Starving the body for a couple of days turns off the gene for PKA, and this is the trigger that tells your stem cells to shift into regeneration mode. According to Valter Longo, professor of gerontology and biological sciences at the University of Southern California, this is what 'gives the OK for stem cells to go ahead and begin proliferating and rebuild the entire system'. Fasting for three days also led to a reduction of IGF-1, a growth factor hormone linked to aging, cancer, and tumor growth. According to co-author Tanya Dorff: '*The results of this study suggest that fasting may mitigate some of the harmful effects of chemotherapy.*"

(http://fitness.mercola.com/sites/fitness/archive/ 2014/06/20/eating-breakfast-intermittent-fasting.aspx; December/2014).

Adaptogens

Before we leave the healing plants field, I need to bring to your attention a group of plants created by God to protect the body from harmful substances.

Numerous studies show that some plants have the power to nourish and protect the body at the same time, helping it to coope and adapt to any stressful situation; they are called adaptogens.

The definition of *adaptogen* is 'a new class of metabolic regulators (of a natural origin) which increase the ability of an organism to adapt to environmental factors and to avoid damage from such factors'.

'This class of herbs is frequently used as a unique and natural alternative medicine and herbal remedy for treating the many forms of stress we encounter in our daily life and the widespread stress-related complications we fall victim to. Adaptogen herbs are non-toxic and essentially have few if any side effects on either physical or mental health.'(http://www.essenceofstressrelief.com/adaptogenic-herbs.html ;December/2014).

The most known adaptogenic plants are the following:

- dragon herb(*Schisandra chinensis*)
- *jiaogulan* (*Gynostemma pentaphyllum*)
- *gotu kola* (*Centella asiatica*) (I took this)
- amalaki (*Emblica officinalis*)
- ashwagandha (*Withania somnifera*)
- *eleuthero* (*Eleutherococcus senticosus*), or Siberian ginseng
- ginseng (*Panax ginseng*)
- *guduchi* (*Tinospora cordifolia*)
- *haritaki* (*Terminalia chebula*)
- long pepper (*Piper longum*)
- rhodiola (*Rhodiola rosea*)
- *shatavari* (*Asparagus racemosus*)
- tulsi (*Ocimum sanctum*)
- licorice (*Glycyrrhiza glabra, G. uralensis*).

For more information on adaptogenic plants, see http://organicindiausa. com/article-adaptogens-the-best-overall-herbs/.

I mentioned those plants here because, of all the herbs studied and used throughout the world, adaptogenic herbs are the most effective in reducing stress and preventing many of its harmful consequences. I personally have used Gotu kola two pills a day.

It is very important to learn about plants' healing power, as they hold the key to our health. Our ancestors possessed that knowledge more than we do today due to the increased trust and consideration accorded by humans to the technology and chemicals which bring them more profit.

Most of the plants contain *phytochemicals*, but some of them have a big percentage.

Recent reports have demonstrated the antioxidant, anti-inflammatory, anti-proliferative and pro-apoptotic effects of various phytochemicals altering the activity and/or expression of some cell adhesion molecules that are mainly responsible for cancer promotion.

Moreover, the pro-apoptotic and anti-proliferative effects of phytochemicals indicate their ability to inhibit the growth of several types of cancers of the blood, skin, brain, colon, ovaries, breast, prostate, and pancreas.

There are many naturally occurring phytochemicals present in foods such as vegetables, fruits, spices, and plant roots, which can kill cancer cells.

Let's remember some of them.

> The anti-cancer effect of **Curcumin** [extracted from Tumeric, presented above] results from its ability to inhibit tumour growth and metastasis. Curcumin and its derivatives inhibit the proliferation of breast cancer (BC) cell lines and induce apoptosis. In the BC cell line MDA-MB-231, cellular proliferation was inhibited via down-regulation of the expression of the cell cycle regulator cyclin D and NF-κB.

Isoflavone (**Genistein**), a naturally occurring chemical in soybeans, has a protective effect against localized prostate cancer, non-small cell lung cancer, and oestrogen and progesterone receptor positive (ER+, PR+) breast tumours. Using similar mechanisms to that of Curcumin, Genistein sensitizes cancer cells to chemotherapeutic drugs and induces breast, pancreatic and prostate cancer cell death by promoting the expression of pro-apoptotic proteins, inactivating NF-κB, and inducing cell cycle arrest.

Indol-3-Carbinol (I3C), extracted from cruciferous plants, plays an important role in inhibiting carcinogenesis by protecting cells from oxidative stress. The chemical derivative of I3C, 1-Benzyl-indole-3-carbinol has a 1000 fold higher activity than I3C in inhibiting the growth of both oestrogen-dependent and -independent breast tumours.

In a recent study, extract from the blue green algae **Spirulina platensis**, combined with selenium (an element with anti-cancer activity), was shown to inhibit the growth of MCF7 BC cell line. This combination is believed to induce cell cycle arrest at G1 stage by inhibiting cyclin dependent kinases. The active compound of these extracts, C-phycocyanin (C-PC) is a water-soluble biliprotein that has anti-inflammatory and anti-oxidant effects and has been reported to induce apoptosis in MCF7 breast cancer cells.

Grape seed extract contains **Resveratrol** (RE) that inhibits cancer cell proliferation by triggering cell cycle arrest through cell cycle regulatory proteins such as cyclin E and cyclin D1. Furthermore, resveratrol induces apoptosis by up-regulating the expression of tumor suppressor genes p21Cip1/WAF1, p53, the pro-apoptotic protein Bax, activating Caspase apoptotic signals, and down-regulating the expression of the anti-apoptotic proteins Bcl-2, Bcl-X$_L$ was demonstrated that resveratrol synergizes with Indole 3 Carbinol to inhibit proliferation and survival of ovarian cancer cells, by down regulating SVV.

Quercetin is a plant-derived flavonoid present in fruits, vegetables and tea. Quercetin induces cell apoptosis through a multi-targeting mechanism by inducing the expression of Bax and activating TRAIL-induced apoptosis. Quercetin also suppresses the activity of Bcl-2 protein family and induces the DNA fragmentation process.

(http://www.jcancer.org/v04p0703.htm December 2014).

***Amla* or *amlaka*(*Emblica officinalis*)** is one of the most common ancient Ayurvedic medicines commonly used to treat a variety of disorders related to the digestive system, the lungs, metabolism, bleeding, and even cancer.

The amla is the fruit of *Phyllanthus emblica*, also called *Emblica officinalis*. The plant, a member of the Euphorbiaceae family, is found growing in the plains and submountain regions all over the Indian subcontinent from sea level to the foothills of the Himalayan mountains.

The fruit is similar in appearance to the common gooseberry (*Ribes spp.*, a type of currant), which is botanically unrelated to Amla. However, due to the similar appearance of the fruit clusters, Amla is usually called the 'Indian gooseberry.'

When the fruit is dried, the main ingredient, water, is mostly eliminated, and the remaining constituents include roughly:

Carbohydrates 70–75% (fiber, about 17% and sugars/starches/gums, about 25%) Polyphenols: 28%

Minerals: 4–6% (calcium, magnesium, potassium, sodium, zinc, iron, etc.)

Miscellaneous other components: 2.5–3.5%(gallic acid, ellagic acid)

Protein: 2.5–3.5%

Fats 1.5–2.0%

Residual moisture: 6–9%'

(http://www.truthorfiction.com/rumors/j/johnshop kinscancer.htm December/2014).

Herb Robert (*Geranium robertianum*) is an enigmatic herb with a miraculous action in tumour diseases, managing to stop or even cure some cancers; it can also boost the immune system. The healing constituents of this herb are found in the stems, leaves, and roots; it has a wide range of healing properties due to its astringent, antibiotic, antiseptic, antiviral, and anti-inflammatory agents.

'Geranium Robertianum is a good source of germanium, an essential mineral needed for the transport of oxygen to the cells. Germanium also promotes electrical activity within the cells, provides energy and strengthens the immune system. This mineral helps provide the antioxidant properties that make the herb such an effective healing remedy. Geranium Robertianum also contains other vital minerals, including iron, calcium, magnesium, potassium, and phosphorus, in addition to vitamins A, B, and C. It also contains the tannins believed to be responsible for the astringent action and ability of the herb to sooth toothaches, sore throats, and mouth ulcers.'(http://www.wisegeek.com/what-are-the-medical-uses-of-geranium-robertianum.htm ; March 2015).

Geranium robertianum is a popular tonic with a strong nutritional content and powerful antioxidant action. Drinking this elixir will help relieve the symptoms of many afflictions. There are studies showing that *Geranium robertianum* can also help people who are suffering from chronic fatigue.

> Drinking tea made from the boiled leaves of Geranium Robertianum can heal gastrointestinal disorders including inflammation and peptic ulcers. The tea has also been used as a remedy for other diverse conditions as typhoid, tuberculosis, boils, malaria, and infections of the urinary tract. A dilution of the tea can be used as an eye wash to reduce inflammation of the eye.
>
> The ability of Geranium Robertianum to increase the amount of oxygen in the cells has caused some to use it as a remedy for cancer. Since cancer cannot thrive in an oxygen-rich environment, it is believed that herb Robert can decrease the amount of cancer cells and shrink the tumours. (http://www.wisegeek.com/what-are-the-medical-uses-of-geranium-robertianum.htm March 2015)

Two years ago, I met a naturopath in Melbourne who cured herself from breast cancer using mostly herb Robert, and she gave me a pot with the plant. Unfortunately, I lost her name.

Also I found the plant growing naturally at the Sassafras Reserve in Dandenong mountains, near the natural spring, growing in great harmony with the *Urtica dioica* (sting nettle), another great tonic for the blood.

Another plant used in cancer treatment is *Pau d'Arco*. Tea made from Pau d'Arco is thought to have been used by the ancient Incas and natives of the South American rainforests, who took it to cure diseases and as a tonic to strengthen the body and improve overall health.

Pau d'Arco((*Tabebuia avellanedae*) contains at least twenty active compounds, such as naphthaquinones (of which lapachol is antitumoral), anthroquinones, quercetin, and other flavonoids whose effects are not fully known.

'In lab studies, lapachol has shown to have great potential of application in fighting metastasis. According to Dr. David Boothman, a professor at the Harold C. Simmons Comprehensive Cancer Center and senior author of a study that appeared in the Proceedings of the National Academy of Sciences, beta-lapachone disrupts the cancer cell's ability to repair its DNA, ultimately leading to the cell's demise. Beta-lapachone and lapachol have also been found effective in killing certain types of bacteria, fungi, viruses, and parasites as well as possessing anti-inflammatory properties.' (http://www.exhibithealth.com/natural-knowledge-base/health-benefits-of-pau-darco-tea-516/ March 2015).

In its isolated form, lapachol is quite aggressive, but in Pau d'Arco tea, nature has brought together a concert of healing substances in the inner bark, which acts in a synergistic manner. It should in no way be limited to any individually extracted substance.

Read more at 'Health Benefits of Pau d'Arco Tea', on http://www.exhibithealth.com/natural-knowledge-base/health-benefits-of-pau-darco-tea-516/. March 2015)

Soursop, Graviola (*Annona muricata*)

One alternative treatment of cancer that has been used in the past, especially in countries where it grows well, is Soursop (*Annona muricata* or graviola).

> Graviola is an evergreen tree native to tropical regions and its fruit and leaves are treating cancer more effectively than chemotherapy drugs without having the same undesirable side effects.

> On the market you can find an extract called Triamazon but the product is not accepted in all countries due to the potential profit loss for pharmaceutical companies.

> 'Graviola is not just a cancer treatment, it has also displayed anti-parasitic, antimicrobial, anti-inflammatory, antirheumatic, painkiller and cytotoxic

properties, according to Memorial Sloan-Kettering Cancer Centre.

In an assessment of Graviola, published in the December 2008 issue of the 'Journal of Dietary Supplements' by U. S. researchers Lana Dvorkin-Camiel and Julia S. Whelan, multiple in-vitro studies determined that the plant is effective against various microbial and parasitic agents. Graviola displayed specific effectiveness on parasites: Leishmania braziliensis, Leishmania panamensis, Nippostrongylus braziliensis, Artemia salina and Trichomonas vaginalis, as well as against the Herpes simplex virus.

As it relates directly to cancer, test-tube and animal research demonstrates that Annona Muricata may be an anti-cancer agent, according to the Memorial Sloan-Kettering Cancer Center, MSKCC. The extract proved to be effective against liver cancer and breast cancer cells. Naturopath Leslie Taylor, author of 'The Healing Power of Rainforest Herbs,' notes that studies shows Graviola has an inhibitory effect on enzyme processes in some cancer cell membranes and only affected cancer cell membranes and not those of healthy cells. This research may lend support to the herb's traditional use against cancer.

Research done over 20 laboratory tests by one of America's largest drug manufacturers suggests that the extracts were able to demonstrate the following:

- Effectively target and kill malignant cells in 12 types of cancer, including colon, breast, prostate, lung and pancreatic cancer.
- The tree compounds proved to be up to 10,000 times stronger in slowing the growth of cancer cells than Adriamycin, a commonly used chemotherapeutic drug

- What's more, unlike chemotherapy, the compound extracted from the Graviola tree selectively hunts down and kills only cancer cells. It does not harm healthy cells.(http://www.jsscon.org/ejournal/articals/artical26.html;March 2015).

Turkey tail (Coriolus Versicolor) also known as the turkey-tail mushroom, contains large quantities of Beta-glucans that act to stimulate the immune system. Coriolus can dramatically regenerate and rejuvenate the body. Its most active medicinal components are biological response modifiers called protein-bound polysaccharides. These polysaccharides are known as Krestin or PSK in Japan, and as Yun zhi, or PSP in China. There have been reports of cases of Bell's palsy clearing up with use of Coriolus for just a few days. Others have found it effective against bronchitis.

Researchers at the Sloan-Kettering Cancer Center in New York tested several botanicals for their immune enhancing activity, in a study published in September, 2008 in *"Vaccine"*. They found Coriolus versicolor to display the most significant immune activity superior to all other compounds tested. Although the exhibited levels of immune enhancing ability of Astragalus was also impressive, it was surpassed by that of Coriolus.

Japanese researchers screened 200 of the best phytochemicals (plant extracts) known for anti-tumor activity. Coriolus versicolor was designated as exhibiting the greatest amount of anti-tumor activity. In another Japanese study, 185 people with lung cancer at different stages were given radiation. Doctors found those who also took Coriolus showed the best tumor shrinkage and the best survival rate. Another study involving stomach cancer patients produced similar results. Those who received Coriolus survived significantly longer, felt better and had fewer side effects.

Coriolus grows nicely in all of Victoria's forests, on the fallen trees together with many other useful fungus and mushrooms, like *Ganoderma lucidum*, *Cordyceps sinensis*, which I picked up and used (dried and ground in the coffee machine).

Learn more at the following:

http://www.naturalnews.com/025455_coriolus_cancer_supplement.html#ixzz32YBvSA58

http://www.naturalnews.com/025455_coriolus_cancer_supplement.html#ixzz32YAjVNl1

Macassar Kernels *(Brucea javanica)* is a shrub originally from southeast Asia and northern Australia. It is known in Chinese medicinal remedies for its *anticancer properties* and is named *ya tan tze*. It has been subjected to hundreds of studies and clinical trials, all of them aimed to understand better how effective this herb really is and which active constituent gives it its anticancer properties

'B. *javanica* contains alkaloids (brucamarina, yatanina) glycosides/quassionide (brucealin, yatanosid A and B, kozamin, bruceantin, bruceantarin, bruceantinolul) and phenol (brucenol, bruceolic acid). The seeds contain brusatol and brucein. The pulp oil contains fat, oleic acid, linoleic acid, stearic acid and palmitoleic acid. The fruit and leaves contain tannins.' (http://preventdisease.com/news/14/012414_Amazing-Medicinal-Plant-Kills-Malignant-Tumors-and-Destroys-70-Percent-Breast-Cancer-Cells.shtml ;March 2015).

Until now there have been 153 reported compounds in the seeds and aerial parts of *Brucea javanica*. Quassinoids are the main constituents of this species. *Brucea javanica* extract and isolated compounds, specifically quassinoids, show various biological properties and are known for their antitumour effects being selectively toxic to cancer cells and inducing apoptosis.

A study in the *American Journal of Medical Sciences* has shown that treatment with *B. javanica* led to the death of 70 per cent of the cells of breast cancer.

'A recent study aimed to investigate and clarify the effects of *Brucea javanica* active constituents on tumour cells, showed how this herb exerts an impressive efficacy for the treatment of cervical cancer, bladder cancer, pancreatic adenocarcinoma and other several types of cancers where an aqueous extract from this plant was able to cause selective toxicity to cancer cells, increasing significantly the levels of protein P53 (the protein regulating natural programmed cell death).'(http://www.gbpuat-cbsh.ac.in/departments/bi/database/phyto_onco_therapeutic/details.php?id=33 ;March 2015).

For more information, see the following:

http://preventdisease.com/news/12/080812_Surprised-US-Scientists-Find-That-Chemotherapy-Boosts-Cancer-Growth.shtml

http://www.ncbi.nlm.nih.gov/pubmed/19286308

http://www.ncbi.nlm.nih.gov/pubmed/16273300

http://www.healingcancernaturally.com/chemotherapy-useless.html.

Cat's claw (*Uncaria tomentosa*) is a large woody vine that grows in the Amazon rainforest; it gets its name from the spines that grow along the vine, which look like cat's claws.

> Cat's claw was first popularized by the German Scientist Arturo Brell, who in 1926 migrated from Munich to Pozuzo, a small town founded by German colonists in the Peruvian rainforest. Dr. Brell used Cat's claw to treat his rheumatic pain. He later treated another German colonist, Luis Schuler, who had been diagnosed with terminal lung cancer. After other therapies had failed,

Mr. Schuler began consuming cat's claw root tea three times a day. He improved remarkably, and one year later was apparently free of cancer.

Cat's claw is a rich source of phytochemicals: its more than 30 known constituents include at least 17 alkaloids, along with glycosides, tannins, flavonoids, sterol fractions, and other compounds. Scientists previously attributed the efficacy of cat's claw to compounds called oxindole, however, water-soluble cat's claw extracts that do not contain significant amounts of alkaloids were found to possess strong antioxidant and anti-inflammatory effects.

Italian researchers reported in 2001 an in vitro study where cat's claw directly inhibited the growth of cancer cell lines derived from breast cancer, with 90 per cent inhibition.

Swedish researchers have documented in 1998 that the plant inhibited the growth of lymphoma and leukaemia cells in vitro and that cancer patients taking cat's claw along with traditional therapies, such as chemotherapy and radiation, have reported fewer side effects, such as hair loss, weight loss, nausea, and secondary infections.

Reports of clinical trials in Keplinger's observation showed that cat's claw may help restore cellular DNA and prevent cell mutation; it can also prevent the loss of white blood cells and immune cell damage caused by many chemotherapy drugs.

Cat's claw has also showed great capacity to kill viruses, to fight free radicals, and to reduce inflammation'. (http://www.lef.org/magazine/mag2007/mar2007_nu_catsclaw_01.htm.)

I used cat's claw tablets and tincture in combination with other tinctures, like propolis, astragalus, cannabis, etc.

Papaia (*Carica papaya*)

In the old Pacific Island culture, papaia was used to treat many diseases, including cancer.

> The recipe is as follows:
>
> Wash and partly dry several medium-size papaya leaves. Cut them up like cabbage and place them in a saucepan with 2 quarts/litres of water. Bring the water and leaves to the boil and simmer without a lid until the water is reduced by half.
>
> Strain the liquid and bottle in glass containers.
>
> The concentrate will keep in the refrigerator for three to four days. If it becomes cloudy, it should be discarded.
>
> The recommended dosage in the original recipe is 3 Tablespoons/50ml three times a day. It is recommended to read 'Papaya The Medicine Tree' for the interesting stories of 'incurable' people who have used this extract to beat their cancer, and for other medicinal uses of papaya'.(http://www.alagad.com.ph/human-development-and-social-services/3-health/618-papaya-fights-cancer-tumors.html; March 2015).

I presented here only the plants that I used, but there are many other plants with great healing abilities, and if you search on the Internet or books, you can use them too.

About Vitamins and Minerals

For curing cancer, minerals and vitamins are a great help. Your body needs vitamins and minerals so it can perform essential functions, grow and develop, and repair itself.

Vitamins your body needs the most include:

- vitamin A
- thiamin
- riboflavin
- niacin
- vitamin B_6
- vitamin B_{12}
- vitamin C
- vitamin D
- vitamin E
- vitamin K
- folic acid
- pantothenic acid
- biotin.

Minerals your body needs include:

- calcium
- chromium
- copper
- iodine
- iron
- manganese
- magnesium
- potassium
- selenium
- sodium
- zinc.

The top five vitamins which help fight cancer are:

1. Vitamin B_{17}

'Laetrile (i.e. amygdalin) therapy is one of the most popular and best known alternative cancer treatments. It is very simple to use and is very effective if used in high enough doses and if the product is of high quality and if it is combined with an effective cancer diet and key supplements. Laetrile works by targeting and killing cancer cells and building the immune system to fend off future outbreaks of cancer.' (http://www.cancertutor.com/laetrile/ March 2015).

Read Morehttp://www.cancertutor.com/laetrile/

We discussed more about this vitamin at the beginning of this chapter under the title Apoptosis.

2. Vitamin D$_3$

> Vitamin D, the sunshine vitamin, has been recognized for almost 100 years as being essential for bone and skin health. Vitamin D provides an adequate amount of calcium and phosphorus for the normal development and mineralization of a healthy skeleton. Vitamin D made in the skin or ingested in the diet, however, is biologically inactive and activation requires enzymatic conversion (hydroxylation) in the liver and kidney.

> 25-Hydroxyvitamin D is the major circulating form of vitamin D that is the best indicator of vitamin D status. 1,25-dihydroxyvitamin D is the biologically active form of vitamin D. This lipid-soluble hormone interacts with its specific nuclear receptor in the intestine and bone to regulate calcium metabolism. It is now recognized that the vitamin D receptor is also present in most tissues and cells in the body. It regulates cellular growth and influences the modulation of the immune system.

There are observations that suggest that the deficiency of vitamin D associated with living at higher altitudes determine an increased risk of many common deadly cancers.

'Most tissues and cells not only have a vitamin D receptor, but also have the ability to make 1,25-dihydroxyvitamin D. It has been suggested that increasing vitamin D intake or sun exposure increases circulating concentrations of 25-hydroxyvitamin D, which in turn, is metabolized to 1,25-dihydroxyvitamin D(3) in prostate, colon, breast, etc. The local cellular production of 1,25-dihydroxyvitamin D acts in an autocrine fashion to regulate cell growth and decrease the risk of the cells becoming malignant. Therefore, measurement of vitamin D in blood is important not only to monitor vitamin D status for bone health, but also for cancer prevention.' (http://mccordresearch.com/sites/default/files/research/Holick.pdf March 2015).

3. Vitamin C

'One of the most well-researched nutrients, Vitamin C has shown great promise in the fight against cancer, both in prevention and disease-management. Consider a recent study in which forty patients with cancer of the breast, ovary, uterus, or cervix received large doses of ascorbic acid (Vitamin C) and other vitamins.

Another sixty-one patients with other kinds of cancer followed the same regime, while thirty-one patients received no vitamin supplements and served as the control group. The control group lived an average of 5.7 months. Of the others, 80 percent of the patients with cancer of the breast, ovary, uterus, or cervix had a mean survival time of 122 months; patients with other forms of cancer lived an average of 72 months. That translates into a length of life 13 to 21 times longer in those who used vitamin therapy' (http://www.care2.com/greenliving/top-5-vitamins-that-protect-against-cancer.html/1, December 2014).

4. Vitamin B-complex: B_6, B_9, B_{12}, B_{15}

> Vitamin B12 is crucial to life and to general health, being involved in almost every cellular activity in the body. Over 300 enzymatic reactions use this vitamin in some way. Apart from dementia, fatigue and heart problems, some cancers (for example, breast cancer) are known to be associated with lowered levels of this vitamin.
>
> In recent years scientists have become more and more knowledgeable and concerned about Vitamin B-12, particularly for people over the age of 50 and/or those on strict vegetarian diets. Some 72 per cent of vegetarians

are deficient in this vitamin, as it is most readily found in meat.

The vitamin is involved in all aspects of your good health. It is known to help form and regenerate red blood cells. It helps prevent cardiovascular disease by lowering blood levels of homocysteine; it promotes growth and appetite in children, improves brain power, concentration and memory, and is involved in a healthy nervous system. It helps maintain a fatty tissue known as the myelin sheath, surrounding nerve cells. B-12 is also involved in the metabolism of carbohydrates and fats and the synthesis of protein, DNA and RNA.'(http://www.canceractive.com/cancer-active-page-link.aspx?n=513 March 2015).

If you have low vitamin B_{12} levels, avoid taking high doses of vitamin C, which may reduce them further, or add to the vitamin C drip some vitamin B_{12}.

B6-Vitamin: 'this B-Vitamin is essential to maintain a healthy immune system and helps protect the respiratory tract from pollution and infection and also protect against cervical cancer. Vitamin B6 is primarily found in carrots, apples, organ meats, bananas, leafy green vegetables, and sweet potatoes.

In studies, folic acid, also known as folate or vitamin B9, helps protect against cervical cancer and is necessary for the proper formation of the body's own genetic material—DNA and RNA. It is found in beets, cabbage, dark green leafy vegetables, eggs, citrus fruits, and most types of fish.'(http://www.care2.com/greenliving/top-5-vitamins-that-protect-against-cancer.html March 2015)

5. Vitamin E

'In addition to protecting against bowel cancer, Vitamin E works as a powerful antioxidant that reduces the damage caused by ozone and pollutants on the cells. It is found in eggs, wheat germ, liver, unrefined vegetable oils, and dark green vegetables' (http://www.care2.com/greenliving/top-5-vitamins-that-protect-against-cancer.html#ixzz32YGJUf9E, December 2014).

Read more about vitamins at:

http://www.canceractive.com/cancer-active-page-link.aspx?n=513

http://www.care2.com/greenliving/top-5-vitamins-that-protect-against-cancer.html#ixzz32YGJUf9E

http://www.ncbi.nlm.nih.gov/pubmed/16566961.

http://www.care2.com/greenliving/top-5-vitamins-that-protect-against-cancer.html#ixzz32YFlmAe0.

The five most important minerals in cancer treatment are:

1. 'Calcium: A proven protector against colon cancer, this mineral is integral for maintaining the health of bones and teeth, blood clotting, and cellular metabolism. Excellent sources include: <u>nuts</u> and seeds, carrot juice, dark green vegetables, salmon and sardines [and eggs shell—you can grind them and dissolve them in lemon juice].

2. Iodine: This mineral is found in sea vegetables like kelp, dulse, and Celtic sea salt. It helps protect the body from breast cancer and is required for energy and the growth and repair of healthy tissues.

3. Magnesium: This mineral protects against cancer in general by maintaining the pH balance of the blood, as well as aids the formation of the body's genetic material—RNA and DNA. While damaged genetic material can put you at risk for cancer, magnesium helps with to repair it. It is found in many foods, including: nuts, fish, brown rice, whole grains, and green vegetables.

4. Selenium: This mineral helps the body manufacture glutathione, an enzyme required for proper detoxification of the body. Because toxic build-up in the body is linked to cancer, assisting your body with its natural, ongoing detoxification processes helps lessen your risk of cancer. Low dietary levels of selenium have been correlated with higher cancer incidence. Supplementation with selenium is a valuable cancer prevention tool [and a mood enhancer].

5. Zinc: A powerful protective agent against prostate cancer, this mineral is also necessary for the formation of RNA and DNA and a healthy immune system. Zinc is found in pumpkin seeds, sunflower seeds.

Zinc and pectin may inhibit the absorption of Vitamin C, so if you use a combination of those products, take them at least two hours apart. Zinc is also necessarily in vitamin B17 (laetrile) absorption.'(http://www.care2.com/greenliving/5-minerals-for-cancer-prevention.html#ixzz32YFFzkCA; March 2015)

6. Medicinal charcoal : Is used to trap in its pores, the harmful chemicals and toxic products of cancer and to eliminate them from the body. Activated charcoal can also treat poisonings, bile flow, hangover and flatulence and it has a great importance in keeping our body clean from all toxic products derived from the medicine we take and from the intense metabolism of cancer. It is better to take 2 to 4 pills at least half of hour before meals.

Read more about the benefit of minerals at http://www.care2.com/greenliving/5-minerals-for-cancer-prevention.html#ixzz32YFFzkCA.

http://www.webmd.com/vitamins-supplements/ingredientmono-269-activated%20charcoal.aspx?activeingredientid=269&activeingredientname=activated%20charcoal

Physical Activity

When we talk about the body's health, we need to include physical activity as an equally important issue as diet and minerals.

'A growing number of studies have looked at the impact of physical activity on cancer recurrence and long-term survival. Exercise has been shown to improve cardiovascular fitness, muscle strength, fatigue, anxiety, depression, self-esteem, happiness, and several quality of life factors in cancer survivors. At least 20 studies of people with breast, colorectal, prostate, and ovarian cancer have suggested that physically active cancer survivors have a lower risk of cancer recurrence and improved survival compared with those who are inactive. Randomized clinical trials are still needed to better define the impact of exercise on such outcomes.' (http://www.cancer.org/treatment/survivorshipduringandaftertreatment/stayingactive/physical-activity-and-the-cancer-patient March 2015).

'Physical activity is associated with a reduced risk of colon, breast, endometrial, lung, and pancreatic cancer. Randomized controlled trials indicate that exercise affects the metabolism including hormone levels, inflammation, immune function, oxidative stress, increase vitamin D levels and possibly DNA repair capacity.' (http://www.ncbi.nlm.nih.gov/pubmed/22286244 March 2015).

Apart of reducing the risk of cancer, physical activity have many other benefits like:

- helps with the oxygen transport in the body
- improves balance, lower the risk of falls and broken bones

- keeps muscles from wasting due to inactivity
- lowers the risk of heart disease
- lessens the risk of osteoporosis (weak bones that are more likely to break)
- keeps the flow of lymph in the lymphatic system
- improves blood flow to your legs and lowers the risk of blood clots
- makes you less dependent on others for help with normal activities of daily living
- improves your self-esteem
- lowers the risk of being anxious and depressed
- lessens nausea
- improves your ability to keep social contacts
- lessens symptoms of tiredness (fatigue)
- helps you control your weight
- improves your quality of life.

'Too much rest can lead to loss of body function, muscle weakness, and reduced range of motion. So today, many cancer care teams are urging their patients to be as physically active as possible during cancer treatment or after treatment, too.' (http://www.cancer.org/treatment/survivorshipduringandaftertreatment/stayingactive/physical-activity-and-the-cancer-patient ;March 2015).

Depending of your cancer phase, the treatment you have, and your physical abilities, you can do more or less movements. Also you need to keep in mind that there is a great level of fatigue induced by a disease, especially by cancer.

> Treatments such as chemotherapy and radiation therapy can cause fatigue in cancer patients. Fatigue is also a common symptom of some types of cancer. Patients describe fatigue as feeling tired, weak, worn-out, heavy, slow, or that they have no energy or get-up-and-go.

> Fatigue related to cancer is different from fatigue that healthy people feel.

When a healthy person is tired by day-to-day activities, their fatigue can be relieved by sleep and rest. Cancer-related fatigue is different. Cancer patients get tired after less activity than people who do not have cancer. Also, cancer-related fatigue is not completely relieved by sleep and rest and may last for a long time. Fatigue usually decreases after cancer treatment ends, but patients may still feel some fatigue for months or years'.(http://www.ncbi.nlm.nih.gov/pubmedhealth/PMH0032526/ March 2015).

There needs to be a balance between physical activity and rest to offer the right environment for the body to recovery.

You can do easier exercises if you feel tired, but you will feel much better after them; it doesn't matter how small are they. And then you can increase the movements a bit every day.

The easiest exercise is walking for more than thirty minutes in a well-oxygenated area, such as a park or a forest. You can do this daily without spending any money (aside from buying walking shoes and a hat). Walking in the fresh air and sun is more beneficial than exercising in a gym. Do not be afraid of the sun; it has very powerful healing attributes.

'Those who tried to convince the world that the sun, the main source of energy and life to Earth, it is causing cancer, they did this with ill intent to deceive the masses into retreating from the one thing that can help prevent illness,' says Dave Mihalovici, a naturopath and writer.

The truth is that we have been systematically lied to about the sun and skin cancer for years. How many know that there is no definitive proof that the sun—and only it—can cause skin cancer?

Maybe the sun can cure cancer. I have a friend with skin cancer on her nose. She had an operation ten years ago, and since then, she has been walking the dog two times per day, about two hours each time, in the sun, wind, or rain without wearing a hat. She is perfectly healthy; she is eighty years old.

In the book *The Healing Sun*, the author, Dr Richard Hobday, has documented a wide range of studies showing that the sun protects against breast, colon, ovary, and prostate cancer. It can also prevent diabetes, multiple sclerosis, heart diseases, hypertension, osteoporosis, psoriasis, and seasonal affective disorder (SAD).

Then there is the case of Dr Harland G. Call. He was diagnosed with skin cancer and was advised by a surgeon to remove it. Instead, he decided to sunbathe the area where he had cancer

After a short period of continuous sunbaths, the skin cancer has completely disappeared. He returned to his treating physician for confirmation, and his doctor confirmed that the skin cancer was gone and that there was no need for a surgery. Dr Zane R. Kime writes that those who get more sunshine had less cancer and that cancer treatment is helped by sunbathing. Sun exposure can cure cancer by fortifying the immune system and increasing oxygen in tissues. The reality is that the vast majority of people, including doctors, have been misled to believe the myth that the sun is toxic, carcinogenic, and a deadly health hazard.

Therefore, most people subserviently use those toxic sunscreen lotions liberally any time they anticipate direct contact with the sunlight. But really, the most conventional of them are causing cancer.

> The sunscreen industry makes money by selling lotion products that actually contain cancer-causing chemicals [like lead]. It then donates a portion of that money to the cancer industry through non-profit groups like the American Cancer Society which, in turn, run heart-breaking public service ads urging people to use sunscreen to 'prevent cancer'.

The scientific evidence, however, shows quite clearly that sunscreen actually promotes cancer by blocking the body's absorption of ultraviolet radiation, which produces vitamin D in the skin. Vitamin D, as recent studies have shown, prevents up to 77 of ALL cancers (breast cancer, colon cancer, cervical cancer, lung cancer, brain tumours, multiple myeloma . . . you name it). Meanwhile, the toxic chemical ingredients used in most sunscreen products are actually carcinogenic and have never been safety tested or safety approved by the FDA. They get absorbed right through the skin (a porous organ that absorbs most substances it comes into contact with) and enter the bloodstream.

(http://www.naturalnews.com/021902_sunscreen_skin_cancer.html ;March 2015)

The statistics reveal that melanoma skin cancer is increasing despite the flourish of the sunscreen lotions industry.

Dr Auguste Rollier opened the first 'clinic of the sun' in Europe in 1903 at Leysin, Switzerland. He wrote a highly influential book, *Heliotherapy*, and was considered the world's most famous *helioterapeut*.

At the peak of his activities, he set in motion thirty-six clinics. Dr Rollier has embraced the belief that the sun is an unsurpassed drug with a full spectrum. He cured his patients by using a healthy diet combined with the power of the sun.

By 1933 there were over 165 different diseases successfully treated by heliotherapy, including tuberculosis, injuries, rickets, and more. The death of Dr Rollier in 1954 marked the end of solar therapy not because it was ineffective but because it was replaced with 'wonder drugs' from major pharmaceutical companies.

Learn more at:

http://articles.mercola.com/sites/articles/archive/2012/06/04/astaxanthin-as-sunscreen.aspx

http://www.breastcancerfund.org/clear-science/environmental-breast-cancer-links/cosmetics/

http://cebp.aacrjournals.org/content/14/1/227.full

http://www.cancer.org/treatment/survivorshipduringandaftertreatment/
stayingactive/physical-activity-and-the-cancer-patient.

Another good and easy way to exercise is in practising Tai chi.

'Theories of traditional Chinese medicine assert that the body has natural patterns of Qi associated with it that circulate in channels called meridians. Symptoms of various illnesses are often seen as the product of disrupted or unbalanced qi movement through such channels (including blockages), deficiencies or imbalances of qi, in the various Zang Fu organs. Traditional Chinese Medicine seeks to relieve these imbalances by adjusting the flow of qi in the body using a variety of therapeutic techniques'

(http://qi-encyclopedia.com/?article=Qi%20from%20the%20 Wikipedia%20archives December 2014).

Tai Chi, which originated over 2,000 years ago in China, emphasizes breathing and involves a series of movements performed in a slow, focused manner.

'The ancient Chinese described it [chi] as 'life force'. They believed *qi* permeated everything and linked their surroundings together. They likened it to the flow of energy around and through the body, forming a cohesive and functioning unit. By understanding its rhythm and flow they believed they could guide exercises and treatments to provide stability and longevity' (http://qi-encyclopedia.com/?article=Qi%20 from%20the%20Wikipedia%20archives;December 2014.)

> 'Everything in creation is made up of electromagnetic energy vibrating at different frequencies that correspond to sound, light and colour. The existence of electromagnetic fields around every object in the world—known as an **Aura**—is a scientifically proven fact. The Chinese refer to this energy as **'Chi'** (pronounced Ci), the vital life force energy of the Universe, present within every living thing. Western

medical science is now beginning to take a serious look at ancient Far Eastern traditions that focus on Chi, the life force energy which flows through the body pathways—known as **meridians and chakras**—of all living forms, in order to maintain health and wellness, mentally, physically and emotionally.

Chi has been written about and studied for over ten thousand years, from China and Japan to India, the Hawaiian Islands and South America. Chi is the energy of life itself, recognized as the balance of Yin and Yang (male and female, positive and negative, electromagnetic energy), which flows through everything in creation. Chi is at the foundation of many health and fitness practices such as Massage, Yoga, Martial Arts, Reiki, Feng Shui and Acupressure.

The energy of Chi emits vibrant, bright colours (the aura), a vibrational frequency, and a sound. When Chi becomes disturbed, stagnant, imbalanced or depleted, dis-ease and illness begin to take form—the aura becomes darker and discoloured, personal frequency vibrates incorrectly, and the meridians (energy pathways—Chinese origin), and chakras (energy centre—Indian origin), within the body, become blocked.' (http://www.chimachine4u.com/chi.html, March 2015)

'A new study published in Cell Transplantation found that Tai Chi can help raise the numbers of a stem cell—CD34 cells—important to a number of the body's functions and structures' (http://www.huffingtonpost.com/2014/05/29/tai-chi-health-benefits_n_5410470.html).

If you are immobilized in bed and you can't do any movement, you still can practise meditation and 'tapping' until you will feel better.

Tapping involves touching firmly enough with the fingers different points on your body. The most important tapping points are on the sternum, above the eyebrow, under the eye, and on the hands. See a tapping chart at http://www.tappingtosavetheplanet.com/how-to-tap.html.

The thymus is located in the middle of our chests, above our breasts, and is responsible for manufacturing and releasing T-cells, which are an important component of our immune system. T-cells are involved in our overall wellness, helping our bodies to resist *dis*eases like cancer. Overall, the thymus is a major part of our immune system. However, the thymus also creates a connection between mind and body and is sensitive to emotions, stress, and negativity. When we experience high levels of stress, negativity, and an imbalance of emotions, we are more prone to illness.

Thymus tapping is a part of some ancient healing traditions, like qi gong. Practise tapping for a total of five to ten minutes each day for at least one minute at a time.

As you tap, put something positive in your mind. Perhaps incorporate a mantra (e.g. 'I am healthy and balanced'), or express gratitude (e.g. 'I am grateful for my perfect immune system).

Use imagery to strengthen your practice. I really liked to imagine a fairy sprinkling on shining magical dust or brushing out all the cancerous cells. With this image, you can change the colour of the dust to reflect your needs at the particular moment. You can also picture the fairy dust migrating to different parts of the body that might need extra attention. You can also come up with your own imagery. Have fun with it!

Don't tap too hard! You only need gentle tapping to stimulate the thymus gland.

Feel free to incorporate this practice into your meditation practice—while you are taking a break at work, when you wake up in the morning, or at any other time of the day that you feel is right for your body.

To find more information about tapping on the Internet, visit the following:

http://www.tappingtosavetheplanet.com/how-to-tap.html

https://www.youtube.com/watch?v=WhoOhJMTVso

http://www.emofree.com.au/learn-eft/.

As I said at the beginning of this book, we cannot succeed in treating cancer by only using medication and diet. We need to heal emotionally also, and while we keep a healthy diet for the body, we need to have a stress-free 'diet' for the mind too. Otherwise, on the one hand, we may be helping the body by proper diet but, on the other hand, poisoning it by stress and anger.

Let's now explore the magical world of our brain and how we can use it in the healing process

CHAPTER 2

THE MIND

In this chapter, 'we will explore the idea that the brain itself, with its tissue and neurons, that we have until now believed as the source of our thoughts and identity, is actually just a tool, *a receiver of human intelligence and consciousness*, but not its source; and that the human mind is not sourced in the brain any more than the internet can be found in your laptop or your modem'.

(http://www.wakingtimes.com/2015/01/09/nature-mind-holographic-brain/ March 2015).

'Every minute of every day, the billions of cells in our brains send and receive signals that influence everything from the memories we form to the emotions we feel. Upon receiving new information, a nerve cell transmits an electrical signal, triggering the release of chemicals called neurotransmitters trough special connections called synapses. These chemicals act as messengers, passing along instructions that switch nearby cells on or off. The human brain has about *100 billion* neurons and *100 trillion* synapses.(http://www.brainfacts.org/brain-basics/cell-communication/ March 2015).

'What is the real function of our brains? Is it the brain tissue itself that creates our intelligence, or is it the electrical and conductive nature of the brain that allows us to *connect* to intelligence? More or less like a sophisticated antennae, just like Nikola Tesla observed of himself early in the 20th century.' (http://www.wakingtimes.com/2015/01/09/nature-mind-holographic-brain/ March 2015).

'My brain is only a receiver. In the Universe there is a core from which we obtain knowledge, strength and inspiration. I have not penetrated into the secrets of this core, but I know that it exists' (Nikola Tesla).

There are numerous research conducted in the fascinating world of our brain function, starting from Descartes and Hippocrates until now in modern times.

We can look at Dr Wilder Penfield's experiments presented in his lectures (*The Mechanism of Memory,* and *Some Mechanisms of Consciousness Discovered During Electrical Stimulation of the Brain*) or at Dr Eileen P. G. Vining of JHU, who studied fifty-four children who underwent the operation.

> And she was simply astounded by the 'retention of memory, and by the retention of the child's personality and sense of humour.' A new version of the study was published in 2003 by John Hopkins University that dealt with 111 kids who had the operation between 1975 and 2003. Out of these 111 children 86% of them were seizure free or no longer needed medication (David Wilcock, *The Source Field Investigations*).

> If memories are stored in the brain, then after this operation those children should have lost those memories pertaining to the removed portion of their brain . . . if memories are stored in the brain. Yet the results were astonishing, and once again defied conventional thought.'

> (http://www.wakingtimes.com/2014/07/01/brain-exploring-nature-mind-holographic-brain/ March 2015).

Dr John Lorber is one of the world's top experts on the condition known as hydrocephalus.

> Hydrocephalus is due to a problem with the flow cerebral spinal fluid which surrounds and cushions the brain, and when there is a blockage in this flow the pressure within the individual's cranium is increased. Hydrocephalus means literally 'water on the brain', and brain swelling in this case leads to a dramatic compression of brain tissue.

> Dr. Lorber studied a total of **253 people** with this condition. In the most severe cases, the pressure in the brain would increase to such a high level that the brain tissue would be compacted leaving the patient with only a fraction of their original amount of brain tissue. In Dr. Lorber's study 9 people reached this severity with around only 5% of their total brain tissue left. That means only 5% of their neurons, brain cells, synapses, and so one were available in the patient's brain.

> 'Amazingly 4 out of 9 of those people with less than 5% of their brain tissue had an IQ over 100, and 2/9 had an IQ greater than 126.' In other words 66.6% of them were fine. Given the drastic loss of brain tissue the obvious question is how is this possible? How can someone with almost literally no brain be intelligent at all, above average?

> Dr. Lorber was directed to a student at his university by his peers, literally based on the intriguingly large size of his head, they thought he may be of potential interest. This student had an IQ of 126 and had a 'first-class honours degree in mathematics, and is socially completely normal.'

A brain scan was done on this individual with surprising results. It was found that out of the normal 4.5 cm of brain tissue, his condition had been compressed to only a few millimetres. In other words his head filled with cerebral spinal fluid, and only a few millimetres of brain tissue, yet he was still high functioning with above average intelligence (David Wilcock, _The Source Field Investigations_).

I have no technical understanding of how this is even possible except to simply suggest that possibly the conductivity and crystalline nature of water may be a contributing factor. What those example illustrate, is that we know very little of the <u>true nature</u> of mind, or the brain and that the mind is independent of the brain.

The information discovered shows that all our memories are recorded in their entirety and with the same detail that we experienced them. From where, we do not know . . . yet.

As Johns Hopkins University, and John Lorber's research found, it may not be that our brains are really that important. If children can have half their brains removed and retain their memories and personality, and if people can function with less than 5% of their brain tissue with above average intelligence, then what is the true purpose of the brain but as a _vehicle for intelligence_, not as the source of intelligence?

Our mind is like a highly sophisticated bio-technology that we use to experience this level of reality, <u>create reality</u>, and express ourselves. Like in the movie _Avatar_, maybe we are not actually our bodies but are just operating them.

(http://www.wakingtimes.com/2014/07/01/brain-exploring-nature-mind-holographic-brain/ March 2015).

The question is, are our memories stored in the brain?

> There is actually no evidence to support that and never
> has there been a memory discovered in the brain. This
> is because our brains are constantly changing and are
> not fixed structures.

> If our minds can remember entire songs to perfection or
> orchestral performances, then what is stopping us from
> accessing this on a conscious level?

> It seems that every single detail of our lives is recorded
> with our brain, so the question I have is how do we
> access that information, and from where do we access it?

> The evidence is finally lining up with ancient spiritual
> truths from every culture which expressed explicitly
> that we are divine, and that our true nature is conscious
> awareness, and that we are merely a fragment of that
> divine consciousness expressed in physical form. This
> evidence provides a truly exciting shift in the way
> we can view our minds, and more importantly our
> potential. If an electrode in our brain is able to stimulate
> a vivid recollection, is it not possibly that we can develop
> our imagination and our mental abilities to this point
> naturally so we can use that ability at will?(http://www.
> wakingtimes.com/2014/07/01/brain-exploring-nature-
> mind-holographic-brain/ March 2015).

Just think about the Shaolin monks, who trains themselves to ignore
the emotions and feelings and become able to do things which normal
people can't, breaking the logical limits of a human body resistance.
They teach us how to use the power of the mind over the body.

'Is it not possible that there is much more going on during a simple
thought process or recollection of an event than we give ourselves credit
for? That is exactly what Wilder Penfield found which caused him at

the end of his career to see the nature of mind as a field of energy which Deepak Chopra called later the "mind-field".'

(http://www.wakingtimes.com/2014/07/01/brain-exploring-nature-mind-holographic-brain/ March 2015).

I presented those studies here because I wish you to understand that your brain is like a notebook in which you can write your thoughts; it is a tool which you can manipulate to heal.

Remember what I wrote in the introduction: it is your choice to heal and live! Your life is the result of your thoughts. You choose to be a winner or a victim. You have this notebook—your mind—and you can write positive thoughts of healing on it or negative ones. It's up to you.

Just think: what if your essence is not in your brain or in your body, but in a formless field of energy?

'While we often think of our bodies and minds as two distinct entities, it turns out they are much more entwined than we might assume. Researchers are continually finding evidence that the brain has a distinct power to manipulate the body's physiology.'). (https://innerwisdomblogdotcom.wordpress.com/tag/examples/; March 2015)

I wish to mention here only a few examples, but I am sure that you have come across many stories of miraculous healing which had defied all traditional medical knowledge.

1.   Positive Attitude Influence Healing

'For example, in 1989, Dr. David Spiegel of Stanford University conducted a study on 86 women with late stage breast cancer. Half of those women received standard medical care while the other half were given weekly support sessions in addition to the standard medical care. During the sessions the women shared their feelings, talked with other patients, and generally had a positive outlet where they could cope with their illness. At the end of the study, the women in the support group lived twice as long as those not in the group. In 1999, a similar study found that cancer patients who have feelings of helplessness and hopelessness have a lower chance of survival.'(https:// innerwisdomblogdotcom.wordpress.com/tag/examples/ March 2015).

My friend Vasilica with an aggressive breast cancer, was always talking about her death in sentences like 'Let's do this [see this show, do this trip], as I will die soon' or 'I gave all my jewellery to my sister, as I will die soon', and she died in a few months.

Avoid projecting your death on the screen of life; project your health and happiness.

'In recent years, David Seidler, writer of "The King's Speech", claimed to have eliminated his cancer through meditation and imagination. After battling bladder cancer for years and only two weeks away from surgery, Seidler decided to see if he could get rid of the cancer through his imagination. He admittedly thought the idea was a little "woo-woo", but by that point he figured he had nothing to lose. So, he spent the two weeks prior to his surgery envisioning a clean, cream-colored, healthy bladder. When Seidler went in for his pre-surgery biopsy, the doctor was stunned to find a distinct lack of cancer—he even sent the biopsy to four different labs for testing. While Seidler believes his visualization were behind the cancer's disappearance, his doctor labelled it a "spontaneous remission".' (https://innerwisdomblogdotcom. wordpress.com/tag/examples/ March 2015).

In 1964, Norman Cousins was diagnosed with ankylosing spondylitis, a collagen illness that attacks the connective tissues of the body. Doctors told Cousins he had only a 1 in 500 chance of recovering, and that he would have to spend the rest of his life bedridden and heavily medicated with pain killers. Instead, Cousins opted to prescribe his own cure: huge doses of vitamin C and positive emotions. Cousins searched for every funny movie he could find and searched widely for funny jokes. He literally laughed himself well. Eventually Cousins was able to completely reverse his illness. Cousins later documented his story in his book, *'Anatomy Of An Illness'*.

Cousins observes: 'The life force may be the least understood force on earth . . . and human beings are not locked into fixed limitations. The quest for perfectibility is not a presumption or a blasphemy, but the highest manifestation of a great design.'(http://www. healthsearches.org/Categories_of_Q&A/Integrative_&_ Alternative_Medicine/1306_2.php; March 2015.)

A big part of the book *Mind Over Medicine: Scientific Proof You Can Heal Yourself* by Lissa Rankin (Hay House 2013) is about how positive belief, hope, and expectation can trigger self-healing superpowers that manifest physiologically in the body.

If you don't have time to read the book, you can watch one of Lissa's speech at http://www.youtube.com/watch?v=7tu9nJmr4Xs&feature=youtu.be.

2. Thoughts and Intentions Alter the Physical Structure of Water

'Experiments over the past four decades have investigated whether human intention alone affects the properties of water.

Through the 1990s, Dr Masaru Emoto performed a series of experiments observing the physical effect of words, prayers, music, and environment on the crystalline structure of water. Emoto hired photographers to take pictures of water after being exposed to the different variables and subsequently frozen so that they would form crystalline structures. The results were nothing short of remarkable. Now think about the fact that the water is impressed of our thoughts and that our body is 70 per cent water; if we can do that to water, what are we doing to our body when we think negative thoughts?

This question has been around for a while in the alternative medicine realms, because the human body is made up of approximately 70% water. According to the Institute of Noetic Sciences, researchers have suggested that intentionally influenced water can be detected by examining ice crystals formed from samples of that water. Consistent results commonly point to the idea that positive intentions tend to produce symmetric, well-formed, aesthetically pleasing crystals, and negative intentions tend to produce asymmetric, poorly formed and unattractive crystals.

Many people point out that this experiment was a fraud, but it's been conducted multiple times and replicated by some highly respectable individuals in the field of science. The paper I am citing here is from Dean Radin, who has published multiple research papers in peer-reviewed journals. The experiment was conducted at the Institute for Noetic Sciences and Adjunct Faculty in the Department of Psychology at Sonoma State University.

The experiment was done to measure how intention alone affects water crystal formation. Co-Investigators were Masaru Emoto, a Japanese energy scholar and author along with a few other researchers and scientists.

The experiment tested the hypothesis that water exposed to distant intentions affects the aesthetic rating of ice crystals formed from that water. Basically, it tested whether intentions could influence the physical structure of water (as mentioned earlier). Over a period of three days, approximately 2000 people in Austria and Germany focused their intentions towards water samples that were placed inside an electromagnetically shielded room in California. Other samples were located outside of the shielded room so that they could act as a distant control. Ice drops formed from multiple samples of water in different treatment conditions were photographed by a technician. Each image was assessed for aesthetic beauty by over 2,500 independent judges and the results of the data were analysed by individuals who were blind with respect to the treatment conditions.

Results showed that the test was consistent with a number of previous studies suggesting that intention may be able to influence the structure of water.

One of the previously mentioned studies was conducted in the 90's, by Masaru Emoto, co-participant in the study used in this article. He came up with the idea to freeze water and observe it with a microscope. At first, he observed crystals of tap water, river water and lake water. From the tap water he could not get any aesthetically pleasing crystals that were unique in design, not even from rivers or lakes that surrounded big cities. However water from rivers and lakes away from development, produced crystals in which each had its own uniqueness, and were very aesthetically pleasing.

The results from this earlier study (among others) also showed that the shape and physical structure of water crystals changed after giving good words, playing good music and showing, playing or offering pure prayer to the water. Disfigured crystals were also observed when creating the opposite situation.

This also correlates with a study that examined the role of intention and belief on mood while drinking tea. It explored whether drinking tea 'treated' with good intentions by monks would have an effect on mood more so than drinking ordinary tea. The study was done under double-blind, randomized conditions, and results proved positive.' '(http://www.collective-evolution.com/2014/03/08/10-scientific-studies-that-prove-consciousness-can-alter-our-physical-material-world/ March 2015)

'So next time you are feeling negative emotions, or feeling negative thoughts, just remember that you are having a physical impact on your biological system. Your cells, everything that makes up your physical body is always responding to you. So be nice to yourself, give

yourself some love.'(http://www.collective-evolution.com/2013/12/01/
if-thoughts-can-do-this-to-water-imagine-what-they-can-do-to-us/
March 2015).

> Nikola Tesla said it best, *the day science begins to study
> non-physical phenomena, it will make more progress in one
> decade than in all the previous centuries of its existence. To
> understand the true nature of the universe, one must think
> it terms of energy, frequency and vibration.'*

> 'Science works best when in harmony with nature.
> If we put these two together, we can discover great
> technologies that can only come about when the
> consciousness of the planet is ready to embrace them,
> like free energy.'(http://www.collective-evolution.
> com/2014/03/08/10-scientific-studies-that-prove-
> consciousness-can-alter-our-physical-material-world/,
> December 2014)

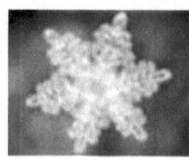

This is a picture of the word *truth* captured in a water crystal. (See more
pictures at http://www.masaru-emoto.net/english/water-crystal.html).

For more details, read 'The Healing Power of Water' by Masaru Emoto
or check the following:

http://www.highexistence.com/water-experiment

http://www.masaru-emoto.net/english/water-crystal.html

http://www.whatthebleep.com/water-crystals/

http://www.collective-evolution.com/2014/03/08/10-scientific-studies-
that-prove-consciousness-can-alter-our-physical-material-world/.

3. The Placebo Effect

'It's been well documented that we can change our biology simply by what we believe to be true.' (http://www.collective-evolution. com/2014/03/08/10-scientific-studies-that-prove-consciousness-can-alter-our-physical-material-world/ ;March 2015).

> 'The placebo effect is defined as the measurable, observable, or felt improvement in health or behaviour not attributable to a medication or invasive treatment that has been administered. It suggests that one can treat various ailments by using the mind to heal. Many studies have shown that the placebo effect (the power of consciousness) is real and highly effective.

> A Baylor School of Medicine study, published in 2002 in the *New England Journal of Medicine,* looked at surgery for patients with severe and debilitating knee pain. Many surgeons know there is no placebo effect in surgery, or so most of them believe. The patients were divided into three groups. The surgeons shaved the damaged cartilage in the knee of one group. For the second group they flushed out the knee joint, removing all of the material believed to be causing inflammation. Both of these processes are the standard surgeries people go through who have severe arthritic knees. The third group received a 'fake' surgery, the patients were only sedated and tricked that they actually had the knee surgery. For the patients not really receiving the surgery, the doctors made the incisions and splashed salt water on the knee as they would in normal surgery. They then sewed up the incisions like the real thing and the process was complete. All three groups went through the same rehab process, and the results were astonishing. The placebo group improved just as much as the other two groups who had surgery.

Another great example of the placebo effect came from the United States Department of Health and Human Services in 1999. The report discovered that half of severely depressed patients taking drugs improve compared to the thirty-two percent taking a placebo. Don't forget about all of the side effects and dangers that have been associated with antidepressants every year. Don't forget that the 'depression industry' alone is a multi-billion dollar one.

A 2002 article published in the American Psychological Association's *prevention & treatment*, by University of Connecticut psychology professor Irving Kirsch titled, 'The Emperor's New Drugs,' made some more shocking discoveries. He found that 80 percent of the effect of antidepressants, as measured in clinical trials, could be attributed to the placebo effect. This professor even had to file a Freedom of Information Act (FOIA) request to get information on the clinical trials of the top antidepressants.

Researchers all over the world have found that placebo treatments can stimulate real biological and physiological responses. Everything from changes in heart rate to blood pressure and even chemical activity in the brain. It's been effective with a number of different ailments from arthritis, depression, fatigue, anxiety, Parkinson's and more.

So what does this mean?

It means that through the power of belief, your biological body can react in a necessary way to target whatever ailment you are experiencing. Thoughts, feelings, and emotions are directly responsible for changing your biology. If we look at depression for example, we are told the main cause of it is a chemical deficit in the brain. But if thoughts, feelings and emotions can release different chemicals in the brain, why not just work on the patients feelings to induce a different chemical state? If our feelings, emotions and thoughts are directly correlated with our biology, why aren't we putting more resources into this research? Why is this not practiced by the medical industry? Why do we completely turn a blind eye to it?

The human race has been trained, and programmed to believe that external medicines are necessary for all ailments. I'm not saying that some medical applications are not valid, I'm just saying the human race completely ignores the power of non-physical phenomenon. We continue to believe that we need something outside of ourselves to heal, when everything points to the fact that this is not entirely true. Our own biological system and the human being is very capable of healing itself. We just don't know how, we don't believe it, we are not exposed to it.

Changing your biology with belief is not an easy process, because most of us don't truly believe we can. We are going up against years of perceptual manipulation that have formed our thoughts and beliefs. Your beliefs shape your perception, and your perception is what creates real phenomenon. If you change the way you perceive things, the things you perceive change. We are powerful beings, and have abilities that have yet to be unlocked. I believe that these types of realities will continue to emerge and will be implemented in the future. The placebo effect demonstrates, from a biological standpoint, that what you believe indeed becomes your reality. For one to be able to use this, they must believe it. One must perceive it as real as the perceive their own hand real, the sun real, the stars real. It's not about believing, it's about knowing.

The true nature of reality has yet to be discovered, but we continue to progress in our understanding. As we progress we realize how obsolete our current way of functioning really is. It's time to evolve past our archaic ideas and false beliefs, and step into a new understanding of reality. We are capable of so much more, or potential is limitless'. (http://www.collective-evolution.com/2013/07/21/the-placebo-effect-transforming-biology-with-belief/#sthash.rDzq0iaM.dpuf)

'One of the most compelling examples of the mind's impact on the body can be witnessed in scientific laboratories across the world. Researchers conducting experiments with sub-atomic particles have found that the molecules actually behave differently if they are being watched. Think about this phenomenon. If a person can influence how subatomic particles behave by just passively watching them, imagine what effect a person can have by actively concentrating on the particles. This phenomenon holds true for every cell of your body. Your thoughts, emotions, fears, and anxieties change the chemistry of your body.'

(http://www.healthsearches.org/Categories_of_Q&A/Integrative_&_ Alternative_Medicine/1306_2.php;March 2015).

A very powerful example to support this affirmation is meditation.

Meditation

A group of Harvard neuroscientists interested in mindfulness meditation have reported that brain structures change after only eight weeks of meditation practice.

Sara Lazar, Ph.D., the study's senior author, said in a press release:

'Although the practice of meditation is associated with a sense of peacefulness and physical relaxation, practitioners have long claimed that meditation also provides cognitive and psychological benefits that persist throughout the day.'

To test their idea the neuroscientists enrolled 16 people in an eight-week mindfulness-based stress reduction course. The course promised to improve participants' mindfulness and well-being, and reduce their levels of stress.

Everyone received audio recordings containing 45-minute guided mindfulness exercises (body scan, yoga, and sitting meditation) that they were instructed to practice daily at home. And to facilitate the integration of mindfulness into daily life, they were also taught to practice mindfulness informally in everyday activities such as eating, walking, washing the dishes, taking a shower, and so on. On average, the meditation group participants spent an average of 27 minutes a day practicing some form of mindfulness.

Magnetic resonance images (MRI scans) of everyone's brains were taken before and after they completed the meditation training, and a control group of people who didn't do any mindfulness training also had their brains scanned. After completing the mindfulness course, all participants reported significant improvement in measures of mindfulness, such as *'acting with awareness'* and *'non-judging.'*

What was startling was that the MRI scans showed that mindfulness groups increased grey matter concentration within the left hippocampus, the posterior cingulate cortex, the temporo-parietal junction, and the cerebellum; brain regions involved in learning and memory, emotion regulation, sense of self, and perspective taking!

Britta Hölzel, the lead author on the paper says:

'It is fascinating to see the brain's plasticity and that, by practicing meditation, we can play an active role in

changing the brain and can increase our well-being and quality of life.'

Sarah Lazar also noted,

'This study demonstrates that changes in brain structure may underlie some of these reported improvements and that people are not just feeling better because they are spending time relaxing.'

'There are some basic, fundamental differences among the kinds of meditation that most people practice, and these differences ought to be considered while you're deciding what is right for you. Please keep in mind that meditation is like food for the spirit: any kind of food is better than nothing. But certain kinds of foods are better than others, and though everyone must to some extent find out what is right for their own body, there are some constant features of food that will have much the same effect on everyone.'(http://www.meditationcenterofthetreasurecoast. com/ March 2015).

There are many types of meditation. The best classification which I found was made by Dr Asatar Bair on his website http://meditation2point0. com/blog/8-basic-kinds-meditation-and-why-you-should-meditate-your-heart.

This is his classification (excepting the prayer):

1. Prayer is the most practiced and common type of meditation. You meditate/think of your needs and actions, ask forgiveness, and forgive whoever has trespassed you. Conform to Catherine Ponder's book *The Prospering Power of Prayer*. There are four types of prayers: general prayer, prayer of denial, prayer of affirmation, and prayer of silence/meditation.

    The general prayer is the act of praying to God as a loving, caring Father in your own way or using the Lord's Prayer, calling upon the God's name (Jehovah) or the Son's name (Jesus Christ).

The prayers of denial will help you to refuse accepting things as they are, to dissolve your negative thoughts about them, and to clear up old conditions of the past. Here is an example of denial prayer: 'I dissolve in my mind and in the minds of all others any idea that my own good can be withheld from me. That which is for my highest good now comes to me through God's grace, and I welcome it.'

The prayer of affirmations is uplifting giving you hope. Here is an example of an affirmation prayer: 'I trust that the power of God which overpass all understandings will bring in my life only the good and right things for me.'

If you are a religious person, use the payer as a meditation and connect with a higher power or God, asking for healing and help to understand what this disease is meant to bring to the surface in your life, what emotions and past mistakes you need to clean and forgive.

As for silence/contemplation, it is said that when you manage to silence your thoughts, you will hear the voice of God. You can find the beauty and bliss of God just by sitting on top of a hill and watching the union of the sky with the mountains and the forest in a marvellous dance of oneness. In that moment of silence and gratitude, you realize the infinite love and power of God, and that power and love will fill your heart giving you faith and hope.

2. Mindfulness, 'also called "Vipassana", comes from the Buddhist tradition. It's all about 'being present', letting your mind run, and accepting whatever thoughts come up, while practicing detachment from each thought. Mindfulness is taught along with an awareness on the breath, though the breathing is often considered to be just one sensation among many others, not a particular focus. There is no attempt to change the breathing pattern, which limits this practice and makes it observational rather than active. Changing your breathing changes the energy; just watching what your breathing is doing (particularly if your breathing is shallow, as it generally is) means you are stuck in a low-energy state.'

3. Zazen 'is the generic term for seated meditation in the Buddhist tradition, but in the modern Zen tradition, it is often referred to as 'just sitting'. It is a minimal kind of meditation, done for long periods of time, with little instruction beyond the basics of posture (sit with your back straight). There is no particular attention to the breath, nor an attempt to change the breath. Zazen is the 'anti-method' approach to meditation, but it is often done in conjunction with a concentration on a certain aspect of Buddhist scripture, or a paradoxical sentence, story or question, called a koan. Zazen is very difficult to learn, and it is very difficult to make progress with this method, because of the lack of guidance on how to do the practice. Also, it was developed for a monastic setting, making it difficult to adapt to an active life in the world.'

4. Transcendental meditation 'is a simplified practice that emerges from Vedanta, the meditative tradition within Hinduism. In TM, you sit with your back straight (ideally in the Lotus or half-Lotus posture), and use a mantra, a sacred word that is repeated. Your focus is on rising above all that is impermanent. TM is a more involved method than either mindfulness or zazen. At the more advanced levels, TM focuses on the breath and changes the breath to change one's state of being. TM often leads to leaving the body (indeed, that is the aim of the practice). That is problematic because the energy of the body (and the mind) can be disrupted. Also, the practice is not focused on your life and your purpose, and the philosophy that goes with it is harmful to the heart, considering desires to be 'egoist' and materialistic.'

5. Kundalini is another practice that comes from Vedanta. Kundalini is the name for the rising stream of energy that exists in a human being. The aim of Kundalini meditation is to become aware of that rising stream, and to ride the stream to infinity. The practitioner concentrates on their breath flowing through each of the energy centres of the body, always moving upward, toward the energy center just above the top of the head. Kundalini makes active use of the breath, using breath to move energy upward. Like TM, Kundalini is not heart-based in either its method or philosophy, and

it can have unpleasant side-effects, which happen often enough to have been given a name: <u>Kundalini syndrome</u>.'

6. Qi gong 'is a form of Taoist meditation that uses the breath to circulate energy through the organs and energy centers of the body in an oval pattern called the 'microcosmic orbit'. Attention is focused on the breath and the circulation of energy (called 'qi' or 'chi'). Attention is also focused on the three major centers used in Taoist meditation: a point about two inches below the navel, the center of the chest, and the center of the forehead. Qi gong uses the breath to direct energy, and circulate energy in the body and spirit. There is little sense of how the heart changes and develops, and no connection between the circulation of energy and emotional states, and no core set of teachings on how to work with emotion.'

7. Guided visualization is a popular form of meditation that involves concentration upon an image or imaginary environment. It is usually done while listening to a recording. An example would be to imagine you are in a grassy field, with a clear sky overhead. There is sometimes a focus on the breath, and because the sensation is imaginary, and the impetus for it comes from outside, the practice tends to be rather passive. This kind of meditation does not come from an established meditative tradition like the others listed above, and so it is untested as a method of spiritual development. Not every recorded meditation is an example of guided visualization; the key is whether it contains elements of hypnotic suggestion or the creation of fantasies under the guidance of someone else. If you are listening to a recording where the guide lays out a method for you to do yourself, or calls attention to sensation and energy already occurring within you, that is not guided visualization, but rather meditation instruction. The key is whether you are practicing a method that will enable you to do a practice by yourself or not.'

8. Trance-based practices. The hallmarks of a trance are: awareness of the self and the environment is limited, conscious control of the experience is absent, rational thinking is absent, and memory of the experience is very limited. Often these kinds of practices involve drugs, music, shallow, rapid breathing (which produces

an intoxicating effect), or a form of hypnotic suggestion. Because self-control is so limited, and because of the passivity involved in having a state induced by someone else, a trance state is both potentially dangerous and not helpful for spiritual development. I could've easily not included this as meditation, because it isn't really meditation, but I included it because these kinds of practices are commonly thought to be meditation' as the mind is quieted and you can access higher levels of consciousness.

9. Heart rhythm meditation 'focuses on the breath and heartbeat, making the breath full, deep, rich, rhythmic, and balanced. Attention is focused on the heart as the center of the energetic system. One tries to identify oneself with the heart. By focusing on the breath, you make your breath powerful. And then learning to direct the breath, to feel the circulation of breath as your pulse in different parts of your body, then on your magnetic field, you learn to direct and circulate energy. You are in control of yourself at all times, and you become both more powerful and more sensitive. Further, your power and sensitivity are always in service of your heart, so you become compassionate.'(http://meditation2point0. com/blog/8-basic-kinds-meditation-and-why-you-should-meditate-your-heart).

'So as this list shows, there are some basic differences between meditative methods. Because HRM directs your full, deep, rhythmic breath toward your heart, it has all kinds of positive health effects. HRM is also an incredibly powerful and rapid way of healing the wounds of your heart. HRM is also a powerful way of accessing the state of unity, which is the goal of every kind of meditation. When you meditate on your heartbeat, you access the state of unity in a very unique way: you feel that your heartbeat is the universal heartbeat, the heartbeat of the all life, the heartbeat of God' (quote from the article '8 Basic Kinds of Meditation and Why You Should Meditate on Your Heart' by Asatar Bair found at http://meditation2point0.com/blog/8-basic-kinds-meditation-and-why-you-should-meditate-your-heart;March 2015)

It will bring you in the power of *now*. See details about the technique of connecting with the present moment in Eckhart Tolle's book *The Power of Now*.

For more info on meditation, go to http://www.meditationcenterofthetreasurecoast.com/2013_02_10_ archive.html.

> But the mind's effect on the body is just part of the complex interplay. Your body also influences your mind. Chemical changes at the cellular level impact your emotional state. The simplest example of this is food. When you eat a sugary treat, you feel a temporary rush of energy and euphoria. When your blood sugar level drops soon after, you feel a wave of depression and fatigue. Chemical reactions in your body are driving your emotions.
>
> After you understand how completely interconnected the mind and body are, you begin to recognize that the healing process can never be just about the body or the mind or the spirit—instead, the healing process is a combined effort of all that makes us biological beings and human beings.

Our immune system is affected not only by what happens at the cellular level in the body. Our immune system also is impacted by our thoughts and our general outlook on life. If we are pessimistic about our chances of recovering from cancer, our immune system will not be as potent. Similarly, if we are optimistic about our ability to recover, this positive energy will help strengthen our immune system and aid in our healing'. (http://www.healthsearches.org/Categories_of_Q&A/Integrative_&_ Alternative_Medicine/1306_2.php;March 2015).

Always, having positive thoughts and attitudes can create a positive outcome. The testimonials of other cancer survivors are a great support in being positive about your cancer healing to uplift and encourage us in believing that always there is a way—we just need to find it.

I found the following materials very inspiring and uplifting:

Anita Moorjani's *Dying to Be Me*

http://www.amazon.com/Dying-To-Be-Me-Journey/dp/1401937519

http://www.youtube.com/watch?v=rhcJNJbRJ6U

Dr Lorraine Day's *Cancer Doesn't Scare Me Anymore*

http://www.drday.com/

Jannete Murray Wakelin's *Raw Can Cure Cancer*

http://rawcancure.com/

Dr David Hawkins's *Healing and Recovery*

http://www.amazon.com/David-R.-Hawkins/e/B001H6MLOO

Brandon Bays's *The Journey*

Claude M. Bristol and Harold Sherman's *TNT: The Power within You*

Claude M. Bristol's *The Magic of Believing*

Louise Hay's *Heal Your Body*

Barbara Brennan's *Light Emerging* and *Hands of Light*

http://www.amazon.com/Hands-Light-Healing-Through-Energy/dp/0553345397

Michael Newton's *The Journey of Souls*

http://themindunleashed.org/2013/06/using-your-thoughts-to-better-you.html.

Training to Change Your Thoughts

'Negative thoughts and feelings have a way of popping up at inconvenient times and distracting us from the good things in life. Our minds begin to slide toward negativity more often than on positivity, and dwelling on dark emotions becomes a bad habit that's hard to kick. But, like breaking any other habit, it requires retraining yourself to think in a different way.'

If a negative thought like 'I can't cure my cancer, nothing is working' comes to your mind, you can change it and replace it with a positive one: 'In every day, I am getting better and better, and the cancer is going in remission.' As I said before, it is up to you what you choose to eat, to think, and to do about this cancer.

'When we are stressed we often have a million things happening at once and a chattering mind is one of the last things we need. Therefore, it's very important to be able to spend some time to relax, put things in context and to let go of the old way of thinking and acting.'(http://www.wikihow.com/Let-Go-of-Thoughts-and-Feelings).

Below, are six techniques on making new thoughts pattern, as presented on the website: http://www.wikihow.com/Let-Go-of-Thoughts-and-Feelings).

1. Be in the moment.

'When your thoughts are spinning out of control, what are you normally thinking about? Chances are, you're dwelling on something that happened in the past—even if it just happened last week—or you're obsessing over something that has yet to happen. The key to stopping those thoughts in their tracks is to be aware of the present moment. Noticing what's happening right now, take your thoughts out of those dark corners. This is because very often the thoughts stop just by focusing on them because they are suddenly exposed to scrutiny and your inner desires that are creating the thought process is seen in a different light. It sounds so simple, but as you probably know, it's not always easy to do.

Here is an example of how to stop negative thoughts from bothering you: Look at a nice, positive image. Put a picture with a beautiful landscape in the room where you are sitting the most—or in all rooms. If you look at a calming image, the mind can relax and let go of all the dark burden. This is a good primary method to relax and calm the mind.

To understand the importance of being present, please read *The Power of Now* by Eckhart Tolle.

2. Engage with the world around you.

> Part of the downside of dwelling on negative memories or emotions is that you're forced to be a little distant from what's going on outside your head. When you consciously decide that you're going to come out of your shell and engage with the world, you leave less room in your mind for those niggling thoughts and feelings that normally sap your mental energy. By judging yourself on the theme of those thoughts it can actually make the problem harder to deal with. You might have been thinking about how much you don't like someone then feel guilty or angry for it. This then trains the mind to become habitual or ingrained as a cause and effect process and it becomes harder in future to be in control. Here are a few ways to start engaging on a basic level:
>
> • Be a better listener during conversations. Take time to really absorb what the other person is telling you, instead of half-listening while you worry about other things. Ask questions, share advice, and generally be a good conversationalist.
> • Consider volunteering or otherwise getting involved in your community. You'll meet new people and be exposed to interesting and important topics that may just outweigh the thoughts and feelings you're trying to let go.

- Look down at your body. Pay attention to where you're sitting. Be attuned to your immediate surroundings. Your reality is where you are right now. It's impossible to go back to yesterday, and it's impossible to predict what will happen tomorrow. Keep your thoughts engaged with your physical presence in the current moment.
- Say something mentally or out loud. The physical act of making a sound will pull your thoughts to the present. Say 'This is the present', or 'I am here, living now'. Repeat it until your thoughts are pulled to the present.
- Go outside. Changing your immediate environment can help your thoughts move back to the present as your senses are occupied with expanding to take in more data. Observe the way the world is moving around you, each being living in his or her own present. Focus on small changes, like a bird alighting or a leaf whirling on the sidewalk.

3. Be less self-conscious.

Self-negativity in its wide scope of forms is also the instigator of negative thoughts and feelings for many people. When you're self-conscious, it's as though you have a second reel running through your head, distracting you no matter what else you're doing. For example, when you're talking to someone, you're thinking about how you look, or what impression you're having [on him], instead of fully participating in the conversation.

Or when you are looking in the mirror, don't say, 'I am fat and old.' Say, 'My body has enough resources to overcome disease. I look a bit tired today, but tomorrow I will feel and look better.'

- Practice being more present by doing activities that completely absorb you and make you feel confident in your abilities (your passions, hobbies). For example, if you're good at baking, savour the experience of sifting the dry ingredients, mixing the batter, filling the cake pan, smelling the aroma of your creation as it fills the kitchen, taking the first bite when it's ready.

- When you experience present moment awareness, explore it and remember how it feels, as well as how you got there and recreate it as often as possible. Remember that the only thing keeping you from feeling that freedom in other situations is your own mind, and put aside self-criticism from your daily thought process.

4. Reflect on your achievements.

The world is full of the small joys of helping others, finishing jobs and goals, going outside and seeing a beautiful scene on sunset or enjoying a delightful meal with friends or family. In practice by reflecting on the beautiful aspects of life builds confidence as well as increases your enjoyment of future experiences.

5. Take good care of yourself.

When you're not feeling well, it's difficult to muster the strength and energy to keep yourself feeling optimistic. Do what it takes to keep your mind, body and spirit healthy—those negative thoughts and feelings will be a lot less likely to take hold.

- Get plenty of sleep. When you're running on a sleep deficit, it's difficult to keep your mind functioning in a positive way. Get 7 or 8 hours of sleep every night.
- Eat well. Have a balanced diet full of all the nutrients your brain needs to stay healthy. Make sure you get plenty of fruits and vegetables.
- Exercise regularly. Having a good exercise routine will keep stress at bay as well as helping your body stay in good shape. Both of these effects have a big

influence on the thoughts and feelings that occupy your mind.

6.   Practise visualization.

{Regardless if you are busy or not, you need to find time to relax, visualise and meditate. Visualisation is a very easy way to improve your health. You can close your eyes for a few minutes, anywhere: in a waiting room in a train/tram, in a lunch break at work, etc. You can visualise beautiful places, events or parts of your body which need healing. As an example, try to visualize yourself being healthy and happy, dancing at a party, being free of cancer, and enjoying your life.}

> Or, 'imagine a pleasant, beautiful and grassy field dotted with flowers and other scenic aspects. Take a minute exploring the open space, open blue sky and clean air. Then imagine a city built on the field with towers and buildings, streets and vehicles. Now let the city slowly disappear again, leaving the empty, beautiful field. The relevance of this image is that the field represents that our mind is primarily empty and peaceful, but we have built a city of thoughts and feelings on top of it. Over time we get used to the city and forget that underneath it, the empty field is actually still there. When you let go of them, the buildings go and the field (peace and quiet) returns.'
>
> (http://www.wikihow.com/Let-Go-of-Thoughts-and-Feelings)

'Creative visualization may sound all fuzzy, new age and far-fetched to you.

Many of the world's top athletes use creative visualization to mentally prepare for their sport.

So, if you can put aside your doubts for a moment and give it a try, the results of your creative visualization exercise could surprise and delight you.

Creative visualization involves the use of mental images to project the achievement of a particular task, performance or any desired outcome, like cancer remission.

The key here is the fact that your subconscious mind cannot tell the difference between the images that it is feed during the creative visualization process and reality. As such, perfect outcomes can be created in your own mental lab and used to increase your levels of self-belief and confidence.

Of course the only way that you can "see" for yourself what creative visualization can do for you is to give it a try.'(http://www.wikihow.com/Let-Go-of-Thoughts-and-Feelings).

'Allow yourself to truly feel positive emotions such as joy, pride, excitement during your creative visualization exercise. The strong feelings you experience while performing your visualization exercises raise your vibration to act like a magnet to draw the desired imaged results to you faster.' (http://www.richardaluck.com/videos/creative-visualization-for-beginners/).

If your affirmation or visualization is empty and with no emotion, the result will be the same—empty.

'The brain operates the body based on input from the personality, but the higher intelligence, or subconscious, is the mechanism that controls the body, and that is the soul that we have yet to acknowledge or even begin to understand. That is the free will component that exists long after the body stops. Near-death, paranormal, mysticism, past life memories, and akashic records are now a common thread that drives home the conclusion that there exists a soul within the human body that transcends the human experience and is eternal. As we acknowledge the essence of our soul, we let go of the limitations of the illusion earth-based mentality and reach out to the greater cosmos of life. Many additional realms exist beyond the earth and in other dimensions of time/space. As spiritual beings, we can easily access these places.'(http://www.wakingtimes.com/2014/03/22/brain-create-consciousness/).

Charles Fillmore, in his book *Dynamics for Living*, says, 'Every mental process is generative. From thinking is evolved what is called living. Every thought produces a living organism; Every life expression originated in some thought. All of the detestable thoughts that mankind harbor, produce living organisms after their kind . . .Man is a free agent. He can open his mind to Divine wisdom and know creative law, or he can work out his unfoldment through experimentation . . . The great need for human family is mind control. Mastery is attained through realization of the power of Spirit.'

But what is the spirit?

We will try to get the answer in the next chapter.

CHAPTER 3

THE SPIRIT

In this chapter, we will explore the connection and interaction between mind, body and spirit; how you can influence your health and control your body through the miraculous power of the Spirit.

The results of many researches in this field will come to prove the importance of the holistic approach of our health and the infinite possibilities and qualities of a human being.

How the Human Thought Determines Reality

a) The body as a vibration

> 'Every part of your body vibrates to its own rhythm. Your brain has a unique set of brain waves. In neuroscience, there are five distinct brain wave frequencies, namely Beta, Alpha, Theta, Delta and the lesser known Gamma. Learning mind control at the deeper states of consciousness opens you up to the world of your subconscious mind where you can create your reality at will and with exact precision.

Each frequency, measured in cycles per second (Hz), has its own set of characteristics representing a specific level of brain activity and hence a unique state of consciousness.'

(http://www.mind-your-reality.com/brain_waves. html).

It's said that some frequencies of 432 Hertz and 528 Hertz (the love frequency) are proven to create healing vibrations for the body. The field of sound and vibrational healing is very interesting, and you can explore and use it in your healing.

Also, any type of music which you may like and creates positive feelings for you, it is a great helper in the healing process. I love Andre Rieu's concerts and I found his music very uplifting and of a high quality. You can try it for yourself at : https://www.youtube.com/watch?v=Jy8AtFzfjhg

The following information was collected from the article 'Can We Reprogram Our DNA and Heal Ourselves With Frequency, Vibration & Energy?' written by Christina Sarich and Dylan Charles found at http://www.wakingtimes.com/2014/03/05/reprogram-dna-heal-ourselves-frequency-vibration-energy/).

"There are numerous scientists (not to mention thousands of years of spiritual adepts) who claim light and sound alter our DNA and directly influence our biology. DNA is a type of language, albeit a complex one. Computer simulations and a purely biological approach to understanding the language, have failed however, in the same way that language fails to describe ascended states.

Researchers from the *Gene and Stem Cell Therapy Program at Sydney's Centenary Institute* have proven that 97 percent of human DNA programs, or encodes proteins in our bodies. One of the researchers involved in this study said, '*this discovery, involving what was previously referred to as "junk", opens up a new level of gene expression control . . .*'

This also means there are multiple modalities that mainstream science has yet to give a nod to, which just might re-train or reprogram our DNA—even cells which have become cancerous or are mutilated by the onslaught of *toxins in our environment* and negative emotional baggage which has been proven to have an undesirable impact on health. Many people have compared human DNA to the Internet. It communicates immense amounts of information in microcosmically small, but significant ways, mimicking a vast network of information portals, not unlike the billions of websites connected to one another all over the world. It may account for our *intuition*, spontaneous healing, and a number of other phenomena that *mainstream science* is just beginning to understand.

If you have ever watched a musician who was skilled in playing his or her instrument *technically*, to absolute perfection, but somehow lost the *emotional 'language'*, then you understand that stringing together a perfect phrase or sequence of notes does not account for an entirely separate and subtle language that speaks to the human heart and mind. It is the technical perfection of the right rhythms and notes paired with heart and passion which brings us to our feet. Similarly, DNA can be *strung together* in its typical set of A-T or C-G, but it is the junk DNA which might decide whether your cells cause you to *develop cancer* or be gifted with the ability to see clairvoyantly.

Russian linguists, Dr. Pjotr Garajajev and Vladimir Poponin *found* that DNA does *follow similar patterns and rules to human language*, but this is not the most interesting information. In fact, biologist, Dr. David Deamer and Susan Alexjander, who holds an MA in music, have discovered that *DNA makes its own beautiful music* before we even try to alter it. The two measured the actual molecular vibrations of DNA and recorded it using an infrared spectrophotometer. They exposed each section of DNA to infrared light and measured the wavelength it absorbed, and therefore determined its sound frequency. What it made was 'hauntingly beautiful' music. 'Some of the combinations of frequencies,' Alexjander said: 'they are just stunning. It sounds alive to me.'

Science does, however confirm that sound and light can and do directly influence the body' healing processes. *Researchers at the University of Cincinatti* have had measurable success in applying high-frequency electrical signals to vascular cells with great effect in healing chronic, persistent wounds like diabetic ulcers. For decades the mystery of Royal Rife and his frequency healing machines have been touted by many as the end-all cure for a wide array of diseases, parasites, and bacterial and fungal infections. His discoveries suggest that every living organism has its own unique resonant frequency and that by subjecting the body to electrical currents that target specific pathogens, diseases and ailments can be neutralized and destroyed without pharmaceuticals or invasive procedures. Furthermore, acupuncture, the ancient Chinese system of medicine that works directly with the body's energy conduits and has offered tangible healing benefits to millions over many centuries, has also recently *been validated by scientific research.*

These examples corroborate, to a degree, the ancient spiritual notion that the human body is enlivened by a subtle energetic system that can be manipulated by the application of sound, light and intention. For one to understand this on experiential terms, however, it is necessary to cultivate the sensitivity to detect and direct this energy, but for many, this process of cultivation is simply too demanding and too methodical to be assimilated as a habitual part of daily life. Most people simply do not have the patience and the time in our fast paced environment to achieve the awareness of this.

While science is making exciting advances in understanding our *quantum universe,* the timeless healing modalities of shamanism have of late been forcing their way back into the popular conversation about healing and spiritual development. In fact, shamanism may offer us the best example of how the use of sound and directed energy can bring about healing in the body and psyche.

In a shamanic healer's toolkit, the most commonly utilized and highly prized agents of healing are often Icaros, which are *Sacred songs* sung by the doctor to the patient to affect health and well-being by enchanting the subtle and unseen spiritual influences that may be gripping the body and psyche. In addition to Icaros, shaman will also often employ chacapas, bundled dried leaves, as well as other musical or tuning instruments which create sounds that are influential to the body's energetic system.

Often coupled with the use of *plant medicines*, shamanic practices can have powerfully positive effects on the sick, and some scientists are recognizing that the alkaloid rich medicine *Ayahuasca may be able to assist in curing cancer. Eduardo E. Schenberg of the Federal University of Sao Paulo,* has recently publicized research indicating that the compounds *DMT* and harmine, found in Ayahuasca, have '*been shown to induce the death of some cancer cells and inhibit the proliferation of human carcinoma cells.*'

Similar to the way cancer has been successfully treated with cannabis oil, or vitamin B-17 from the apricot pit, it is emerging as a viable possibility that Ayahuasca is another herbal, ancient cure to this disease found in abundance in the new world of synthetic consumption.

Ayahuasca, is a psychoactive, sacred ancient brew, with deep roots in South American shamanic practice. Since at least 500 BC, South American shamans have used Ayahuasca for ceremonial purposes, and as a medicine of many functions.

Many people believe that DMT is created in the pineal gland of human beings when we dream, when we are born, and when we die. Critics of this theory say there is no evidence to back up these claims, but as of 2013, studies from the University of Michigan have shown that indeed dimethyltryptamine is created in the pineal glands of rats, and with the biological similarities us mammals share, it is very likely that DMT is synthesized in our pineal glands as well. According to Dr. Rick Strassman, author of the critically acclaimed book *DMT - The Spirit Molecule*, the human body metabolizes DMT rapidly, almost eager to consume the substance. Serotonin, the primary source of pleasure for us human beings, created in our brains and bodies daily of course, is 5-hydroxytryptamine, almost chemically identical to dimethyltryptamine. Yet, the US government classifies this molecule that it is part of our very being, highly illegal drug.

DMT is a very complex substance, with complex experiences had by those who consume it, complex origins, and many, many functions. One must do their own hard research on Ayahuasca and DMT. Many of you who have read this far, probably already know what you need to know about Ayahuasca/DMT, as the popularity of it is skyrocketing.

It should be noted that Ayahuasca/DMT has characteristics similar to almost no 'drugs' except perhaps psilocybin mushrooms. Psilocin (what psilocybin metabolizes into), is also almost identical to chemicals already in our brains, similarly metabolized quickly by the body, more characteristic of a vitamin than an intoxicant.

Ayahuasca is a brew consisting of many different psychoactive plants, including dimethyltryptamine containing foliage, and MAOI inhibiting plants that make the DMT active when ingested orally, namely the root bark of the Caapi vine. Caapi root bark contains monoamine oxidase inhibitors, harmala alkaloids. The DMT in Ayahuasca is primarily found in the leaves of the Psychotria Viridis plant, or the seeds of Syrian Rue, or both. Similar to cannabis' ancient, rich history as a medicine, Ayahuasca has been a fundamental part of indigenous cultures in South America, namely the Amazonian rainforest and Peru, for thousands of years.

Ayahuasca is not typically looked at as a tool to treat cancer. More often, people decide to drink Ayahuasca or ingest DMT in pursuit of life-changing experiences, epiphanies, to visit unexplored corners of the mind, in hopes of easing a wide range of psychological ailments and problems and they report extreme mental clarity after the experience, a difficult-to-explain sense of well-being, as if the substances organized the user's subconscious and rarely touched areas of the brain.

While reductionist science is good at isolating molecular reactions, the truth is that any research on the subject of Ayahuasca is incomplete without acknowledging the beneficial presence of shamanic healers who are capable of bringing out the highest energetic potential of the effects of any chemical compounds within Ayahuasca, or any other plant medicine. Administering the compounds without the context of genuine shamanism is hollow, and lacks the full picture of the healing potential of shamanic medicines. The primary means in which shaman communicate with a patient is through their Icaros and other instruments of sound and vibration, which demonstrates their understanding that a significant part of the science of healing is working with *vibration and frequency*.

While certainly an interesting idea to muse, the evidence that frequency and vibration can directly affect DNA and the body's healing processes is still forthcoming [and need further examination].

This is not an easy theory to prove, or disprove, and the answers are unlikely to satisfy everyone.

Certainly, this is a complicated and sometimes heated topic, as we do live in a world still dominated by material science that attempts to reduce mysticism and spirituality to anomalies in brain chemistry and personality. Yet, at the same time, the human race is coming up against serious plateaus in its understanding of how to interact with the natural world, including our bodies, which means we must be willing to tangentially explore the validity of the information received through intuitive experiences.

Miracles happen, not in opposition to nature, but in opposition to what we know of nature' (St Augustine).

It seems that simultaneously with all the other ways we are seeing a global paradigm shift, there is a shift taking place in the realm of medicine. After about a century of criminalizing plants and mind-altering products of the earth, people globally seem to be taking great interest in the Earth's treasure chest of medicine in botany and nature, no longer concealed from us or alleged to be dangerous by proponents of pharmaceutical monopolies. Scientists such as Eduardo Schenberg will surely press on in their work, as the massive surge in popularity for these things grows exponentially.

These questions are here to stay until answered, so aren't they worthy of a second look, with an open mind to *all possibility*?' (http://www.wakingtimes.com/2014/03/05/reprogram-dna-heal-ourselves-frequency-v/ibration-energy/)

You can find more information about sound/vibration healing on:

http://consciouslifenews.com/power-frequency-heal-diseases/

http://jevondangeli.com/tibetan-singing-bowls-the-ancient-brain-entrainment-methodology-for-healing-and-meditation/

http://www.crystalsingingbowls.com/about_crystal_singing_bowls.htm

http://www.wakingtimes.com/2014/01/30/brazilian-scientist-ayahuascadmt-can-effectively-treat-cancer

http://www.wakingtimes.com/2014/03/05/reprogram-dna-heal-ourselves-frequency-vibration-energy/.

b) The body as an energetic structure

The first step is to consider the possibility that we are not only energy, but that there is infinite energy all around us which we can consciously tap into to promote healing in our body and mind, to become a more happy, healthy, vibrant and creative being. As soon as you start to connect to the infinite energy of creation and your own true nature as formless energy, then you start to become aware of these energies in your body which returns the projection of your body to its natural state.

The projection of your body can only be disrupted by a disturbance in your energy field—your consciousness—caused by unbalanced thoughts and emotions, and limiting beliefs.

Our luminous energy field is naturally vibrant, and our energy naturally flows as a powerful stream of consciousness, but the lower levels of consciousness, which we have been conditioned to live in as part of our social indoctrination, disrupt this flow which if left unhindered would express its perfection everywhere.

Another key concept to understand is that your body is *always regenerating.*

[As we learned at the beginning of this book], every year 98% of the atoms in your body are exchanged for 'new' atoms. You are constantly dying, and being reborn, and literally transforming at the atomic and molecular levels. Every three days you have a new stomach lining, every month you have new skin, every three months you have a new skeleton. And every year you have *almost an entirely new body* (Deepak Chopra from *Living Beyond Miracles* with Wayne Dyer).

Deepak Chopra described it beautifully by saying that our atoms 'are like migrating birds'. They are not permanent, they are completely independent, and are drifting through space and time and merely being organized into structures such as our bodies by our energy field which organizes them as a magnetic field organizes metal filings, only slightly more complex.'

(http://www.wakingtimes.com/2014/04/16/proof-human-body-projection-consciousness/

It is well known (especially in Asian tradition) that there are energetic centres, or gateways for the flow of energy, in our body called chackras.

The Chakras System

Our Seven Life Force Energy Centres

'*Chakra*' is a Sanskrit word literally meaning 'wheel'. These centres were named as such because of the circular shape to the spinning energy which exist in our subtle etheric body, the non-material energetic counterpart to our physical body. There are seven main chakras and they are located along the spine extending out the front and back of the body. Each *chakra* has a number of specific qualities that correspond to the refinement of energy from the base-level material-self identity, located at the first chakras, up to the higher vibration spirit-level awareness of being, at our crown. These energetic centres represent our highest level of integration split, prism like, into a spectrum of colors. Our opportunity in studying them is to learn how to master each *chakra's* essence and unite them all into a unified field of brilliance. As such, we re-unite our disparate parts into a radian light of full self-awareness.

The *chakras* are formed at the junction of three connected energy shafts that ascend the spine, one on each side of the central channel, the *Shushumna*. The two lesser channels of energy—the *Pingala* on the right and *Ida* on the left—run parallel to the spinal cord. *Chakras* both take up and collect *prana* (life force energy) and transform and pass on energy. Our material bodies could not exist without them for they serve as gateways for the flow of energy and life into our physical bodies.

Each *chakra* is associated with a certain part of the body and a certain organ which it provides with the energy it needs to function. Additionally, just as every organ in the human body has its equivalent on the mental and spiritual level, so too every *chakra* corresponds to a specific aspect of human behaviour and development.

Our circular spirals of energy differ in size and activity from person to person. They vibrate at different levels relative to the awareness of the individual and their ability to integrate the characteristics of each into their life. The lower *chakras* are associated with fundamental emotions and needs, for the energy here vibrates at a lower frequency and is therefore denser in nature. The finer energies of the upper chakras corresponds to our higher mental and spiritual aspirations and faculties.

The openness and flow of energy through our *chakras* determines our state of health and balance. Knowledge of our energy system empowers us to maintain balance and harmony on the physical, mental and spiritual level. All meditation and yoga systems seek to balance out the energy of the *chakras* by purifying the lower energies and guiding them upwards. Through the use of creating 'internal space', and living consciously with an awareness of how we acquire and spend our energy, we become capable of balancing our life force with our mental, physical and spiritual selves.

In order for us to become fully self-realized and in harmony with our physical and spiritual nature our denser lower energies need to be harmonized with the lighter energies of the upper centres. Indeed, each of the upper-level energies corresponds and refines a lower level counterpart: 7th with 1st, 6th with 2nd, 5th with 3rd. In the centre of our being is full integration into the heart.

Each centre has an integral function in creating our energetic balance. It is through the study of our energetic and physical being that we can create health, emotional stability and spiritual bliss. The following chart maps out the primary qualities of each *chakra*, its corresponding location in the body, colour, physical and emotional realms of influence, and its greater significance.

7	Crown Chakra *Sahasrara* Top of the head Violet Symbol is the thousand-petaled lotus	Spirit Shiva/Consciousness Unification of colours Intelligence/Bliss of Divine Wisdom Pineal gland Upper brain and right eye Gem = Pearl Planet = Pluto Spiral pair = root chakra 7/1 Excessive: cult leader, ego maniac Deficient: no spiritual inspiration/aspiration	This chakra represents the highest level of consciousness and enlightenment. It is the connective centre to spirit. This centre integrates all the chakras with their respective qualities. Mastering the lower vibrational aspects of our being we reside in the full awareness that we are spiritual beings living a human existence
6	Third Eye Chakra *Ajna* Forehead Indigo Seed mantra = *Aum* Symbol is a descending triangle within a circle	Light Knowingness/ Intuition/Perception Self Mastery, wisdom, imagination Pituitary gland, spine, lower brain, left eye, nose and the ears Gem = Diamond Planet = Sun Sense = Sixth sense, higher mind Spiral pair = sacral chakra 6/2 Excessive: overly intellectual; overly analytical Deficient: unclear thought; deluded	The seat of intuition and direct spiritual vision; it is here that we visualize things through our 'third eye' of intuitive knowledge. The opening of the third-eye corresponds with spiritual awakening. It is the chakra of forgiveness and compassion.

| 5 | Throat Chakra *Vishuddha* Throat Light Blue Seed mantra = *Hum* Symbol is a circle within a descending triangle | Ether Communication/ Creativity Sound/Intuition/ Synthesis Self expression/Desire to speak and hear the truth Thyroid gland, throat, upper lungs, arms, digestive track Gem = Sapphire Planet = Saturn Sense = Hearing Spiral pair = solar chakra 5/3 Excessive: willful, controlling, judgmental, hurtful speech Deficient: lacking faith, unable to creatively express, silent child | The center for communication, self-expression and creativity. This is where the inner voice of one's truth is expressed. It is the chakra of diplomacy, of pure relationships with others, and of playful detachment. Speaking with a knowledge of our interconnectivity through Spirit reflects mastery of this energy. |
| 4 | Heart Chakra *Anahata* 'Un-struck' Center of chest Green / Pink Seed mantra = *Yum* Symbol is intertwined descending and ascending triangles | Air Compassion/Love/ open-hearted desire for self-acceptance balance emotions, harmony, place of integration Thymus, heart, liver, lungs, blood circulation Gem = Ruby Planet = Venus Sense = touch Spiral pair = the center 4/4 Excessive: inappropriateemotional expression; poor emotional boundaries Deficient: ruthless, no heart, can't feel emotions | The center of real, unconditional affection, spiritual growth, compassion, devotion and love. It is the bridge connecting the lower and higher energies of our being and is the place where resides our Spirit, our true Self, free and independent. |

| 3 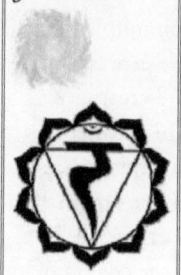 | Solar Plexus Chakra *Manipura* 'Illustrious gem'

Slightly above the naval
Yellow
Seed mantra = *Ram*

Symbol is a descending triangle | Fire Will/Power/Joy/ Motivation self-esteem transformation, identification / mastery will over your own light power in relationship with others vitality, energy standing steady in your own self desire to express individuality Pancreas, stomach, liver, gall-bladder Gem = Emerald Planet = Jupiter Sense = sight Spiral pair = throat chakra 3/5 Excessive: egotistical, self-absorbed; ambitious self-driven warrior, desire to take control Deficient: poor self-worth; sensitive servant; feels disliked; martyr; needing to 'do' all the time | Located at the center of the body it is the place where physical energy is distributed. It is the center for unrefined emotions and personal power. It is the center that give us the sense of complete satisfaction and contentment. Our creativity is fueled by our power of will. |
| 2 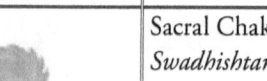
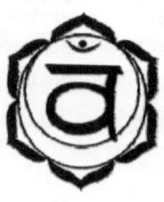 | Sacral Chakra *Swadhishtana*

Slightly below naval
Orange
Seed mantra = *Vam*
Symbol = up-turned crescent | Water Relationships/ Sexuality/Empathy Pleasure/Well-being connection, delight emotions, feeling, polarity, change Gonads and reproductive organs, legs | This energy is the center for creating relationships of all kinds. It is where we develop an inward sense of self and an outward awareness of others, ego, |

		Gem = Amethyst Planet = Mercury Sense = taste Spiral pair = third eye 2/6 Excessive: manipulative, controlling, lustful, addictive Deficient: co-dependent, martyr, submissive, doesn't feel anything, shut down	sexuality, and family and defined as we work with this energy. The feelings of other people are directly perceived through mastery of this chakra's energy.
1	Root Chakra *Muladhara* Base of Spine Red Seed mantra = *Lam* Symbol = Square	Earth Shakti/Manifestation Survival/Grounding/ Stability gravitation drawing into a point trust, survival, self preservation root support, desire to be in the physical world Sense = smell Suprarenal glands, prostate Kidneys, bladder, spine Gem = Coral Planet = Mars Spiral pair = crown chakra 1/7 Excessive: overly possessive; fearful parent Deficient: homeless; ungrounded; victim	The seat of physical vitality and the fundamental urge to survive. It regulates those mechanism which keep the physical body alive. It is the chakra whose main aspect is innocence.

("The Chakras system" by William J. D. Doran -
http://www.expressionsofspirit.com/yoga/chakras.htm)

In a recent interview with Waking Times aired on The People's Voice Network, Dr Eben Alexander, a Harvard neurosurgeon, presented compelling scientific research in the field of consciousness that examines the unfolding reality that the brain does *not* create consciousness.

> Misleading concepts that focus on reductive materialism have kept us in the dark about the true nature of the human soul and its integral part in our evolution as spiritual beings.

> *'The old paradigm of birth to death represents an outdated concept that is woefully inadequate in defining the unfolding reality of expanded awareness,'* he stated in the interview with Waking Times. *'Materialist science is at the end of its days as most scientists are changing their views. The old concepts are soon to be relegated to the same dust bin as 'the earth is flat' as we develop a more mature understanding and transcend old beliefs.'*

> Supported by worldwide research that is now delving into the concepts of string theory that involves a complete reworking of our outdated and limited views of space/time means that we are now entering a phase where science will greatly expand its boundaries. The foundation of the research begins with the clear understanding of the 'Soul', or conscious spirit, that exists outside of the body and is eternal.

> *'Consciousness is at the core to unfolding all of reality',* states Alexander.

Charles Fillmore says in his book *Dynamics for Living*: 'The Consciousness is the sense of awareness, of knowing. It is our knowing that we know . . . It is the composite of ideas, thoughts, emotions, sensations and knowledge that makes up the conscious, subconscious and super conscious phases of mind.'

Dr David Hawkins even created a map of consciousness via muscle testing, on which you can classify every living being in a 'niche' of consciousness.

You can see the image at http://www.pinterest.com/pin/8943874257 2840245/ and read about it at http://personalexcellence.co/blog/map-of-consciousness/.

> 'Edgar Cayce, the father of holistic medicine, pioneered the concept in modern times that we are indeed *spiritual beings having a human experience*,' but this is only a re-emergence of what our ancestors already knew.
>
> This time on earth will be one where we all transcend the false boundaries that convince us that we are separate entities and develop the understanding of the oneness that we all share, meaning that we don't have to be either scientific or spiritual. Merging science and spirituality creates a new foundation for our peaceful coexistence in the greater cosmos'.
>
> (http://www.wakingtimes.com/2014/03/22/brain-create-consciousness/).

The following article, 'Proof That the Human Body Is a Projection of Consciousness' (from http://www.wakingtimes.com/2014/04/16/proof-human-body-projection-consciousness/), explains very beautifully the connection between our thoughts and the manifestation of our reality.

> 'One of the key principles of quantum physics is that our thoughts determine reality. Early in the 1900's they proved this beyond a shadow of a doubt with an experiment called the double slit experiment. They found that the determining factor of the behaviour of energy ('particles') at the quantum level is the awareness of the observer.

For example: electrons under the same conditions would sometimes act like particles, and then at other times they would switch to acting like waves (formless energy), because it was completely dependent on what the observer expected was going to happen. Whatever the observed *believed* would occur is what the quantum field did.

The quantum world is waiting for us to make a decision so that it knows how to behave. That is why quantum physicists have such difficulties in dealing with, explaining, and defining the quantum world. We are truly, in every sense of the word, masters of creation because we decide what manifests out of the field of all-possibility and into form.

The thing is, the quantum level of reality isn't a local and insignificant aspect of creation. *It is all around us,* and it is the most fundamental level of creation aside from the unified field itself. The human energy field is interacting and influencing the quantum field all around us at all times. The energy of our beliefs and intentions are infused into our energy field because they are defined by the energy of our thoughts and emotions.

The human energy field, is perpetually informing the quantum reality within us and around us at each moment of our existence.

And because reality is flashing in and out of existence (hypothetically at Planck time—10^{44} times per second—as explained by The Resonance Project biophysicist William Brown), every time our reality oscillates between form, and the pure energy state of the field, our awareness which is constant and doesn't flash in and out of existence *informs the field what to reappear as* when it makes its transition back to form at the quantum level.

Therefore each time we oscillate into formlessness, we have complete and total control and *responsibility* over what we choose with our attention to manifest out of the field in the next moment, and our power and ability to do so relies entirely on what we believe, and on *how we are feeling*.

A dramatic example of this is the case of Vittorio Michelli. In 1962 he was admitted to the Military Hospital of Verona, Italy with a large tumour on his left hip. The doctors knew that they could not help him, so his case was deemed hopeless and he was sent home without treatment, and after about 10 months his left hip bone had completely disintegrated. As a last resort, he travelled to Lourdes, France and bathed himself in the spring there (which is a Christian holy site famous for producing miracles).

Immediately he started *feeling better*, he regained his appetite, and bathed himself in the spring a few more times before he left. After a few months of being home he felt such a *powerful sense of well-being* that he urged the doctors to x-ray him again, and they were astonished to find that his tumour had shrunk. Over the next several months they kept a close watch on him, and his X-rays showed that his tumour kept on shrinking, until it was gone. And once his tumour disappeared, *his hipbone started regenerating*.

After two months he was walking again, and several years later his hip bone had completely regenerated. The Vatican's Medical Commission, in their official report said:

'A remarkable reconstruction of the iliac bone and cavity has taken place. The X-rays made in 1964, 1965, 1968, and 1969 confirm categorically and without doubt that an unforeseen and even overwhelming bone reconstruction

has taken place of a type unknown in the annals of world medicine.' (The Holographic Universe, p.107)

Ordinarily this would be deemed miraculous, and indeed it truly is. But I find this miraculous in the sense of the true power of human intention and belief that it displays; the power of fate. Moreover, this is powerful evidence that suggests that there is an energetic structure which our 'material bodies' align with, because that is one of the only logical explanations for how Vittorio Michelli's hip bone knew exactly which shape to grow back into, *unless* there was some sort of energetic blueprint which was instructing its growth, which as the Vatican's Medical Commission clearly stated, was *'unknown in the annals of world medicine.'*

In medicine, maybe this was unknown, but the same cannot be said for physics. At the atomic level atoms bond with one another to form molecules which have specific geometric structures as if there is an energetic blueprint which they are adhering to which dictates the shapes they maintain together.

If our bodies are a projection of consciousness, then our consciousness would create an energetic blueprint which our atoms and molecules align with to create our bodies. There is highly suggestive evidence of the existence of this energetic blueprint (or human energy field) in the new research on DNA which proves that it transmits, receives, and thus reads energy directly from the field.

Michelli's case is a perfect example of our human ability to re-organize that vacuum structure with our energy and intentions, and thus manifest what we desire directly out of the field for truly miraculous results. The fact that he started to *feel* better and started to *believe* that he was healed is, the key to his healing.

Some may want to stick with the belief that God healed this man, and I would agree to you. But you and I would probably disagree on the nature of this God. For I contend that you are god, as are we all, because the force we call God is the energy and infinite consciousness behind creation, and thus when we tap into ourselves as pure consciousness, i.e. without thought through meditation, then we open ourselves to the infinitude of our own awareness because we inseparably are that infinite creative consciousness. We are it and it is us.

And when we open up to that energy, we allow ourselves to be flooded with a *'powerful sense of well-being'* and knowing which has astounding power to create reality, and directly affects our biology. (http://www.wakingtimes.com/2014/04/16/proof-human-body-projection-consciousness/).

'A fundamental conclusion of the new physics also acknowledges that the observer creates the reality. As observers, we are personally involved with the creation of our own reality. Physicists are being forced to admit that the universe is a "mental" construction. Pioneering physicist Sir James Jeans wrote: "The stream of knowledge is heading toward a non-mechanical reality; the universe begins to look more like a great thought than like a great machine. Mind no longer appears to be an accidental intruder into the realm of matter, we ought to rather hail it as the creator and governor of the realm of matter. Get over it, and accept the inarguable conclusion. The universe is immaterial-mental and spiritual." (http://www.wakingtimes.com/2014/04/16/proof-human-body-projection-consciousness/)

c) The body as a projection of consciousness

I want you to really understand that reality is a sum of energetic impulses that are flashing in and out.

This is absolutely crucial in understanding our ability to heal, because if half of the time we are formless, then (1) Who are we really, because obviously our bodies and the material world is illusory to a degree; and (2) What is the blueprint which is guiding the rearrangement of our bodies each time we quite literally re-materialize?

The answer to both questions would be Consciousness. Our bodies are a holographic projection of our consciousness, and they are the sum total of our beliefs about ourselves. If we can change our beliefs about ourselves, and thus if we can change the energy that defines our human energy field, then we can *change the energetic blueprint* which our body aligns with as it re-materializes back into form 10^{44} times per second.

(The exact structure and dynamics of our consciousness which make us both a fractal and holographic expression of this infinite God-consciousness can be found in Nassim Haramein's Holofractographic Universe theory, and in his work crossing the Event Horizon.)

Deepak Chopra told a story that illustrates this perfectly in his book, 'How to Know God'. A friend of his, injured his foot while working out in a gym because he was unaccustomed to using one of the machines and strained it. The pain in his foot increased over the next few days, and he found it increasingly difficult to walk, so upon *'medical examination it was found that he had a common ailment known as planar fasciitis, in which the connecting tissue between the heel and the front of the foot had been stretched or torn'* (How to Know God, p. 221).

His friend decided not to have surgery and instead to tough it out, but in time he found it so painful and difficult to walk that he sought out a Chinese Healer in desperation. This Chinese man was ordinary by appearance, and gave 'no evidence of being mystical or spiritual, or in any way gifted in healing'. The injured friend of Deepak Chopra continues:

'After gently feeling my foot, he stood up and made a few signs in the air behind my spine. He never actually touched me, and when I asked what he was doing, he simply said he was turning some switches in my energy field. He did this for a minute or so and then asked me to stand up. I did, and there was no sensation of pain, not the slightest. You have to remember that I had limped in, barely able to walk.'

He continues:

'In complete amazement I asked him what he had done. He told me that the body was an image projected by the mind, and in a state of health the mind keeps this image intact and balanced. However, injury and pain can cause us to withdraw our attention from the affected spot. In that case, the body image starts to deteriorate; its energy patterns become impaired, unhealthy. So the healer restores the correct pattern—this is done instantly, on the spot— after which the patient's own mind takes responsibility for maintaining it that way' (How to Know God, p. 222).

Quantum physics knows that our thoughts and beliefs influence the quantum reality which is the source of the material world. Therefore it is only natural to assume an energetic and formless source for all of creation, including our physicality.

We must start to consider ourselves as more than a physical body; as a luminous energy field organizing ourselves in a body, or as pure consciousness manifesting ourselves and *temporarily experiencing this level of reality through* our bodies. New evidence is clearly illustrating that our mind is non-local and is independent of the brain, which means it doesn't need the brain, or the body for that matter, to exist.

We are so much more than we think we are, and infinitely more than we have been lead to believe. The next step that we have to take, moreover, the next step in our human evolution now involves us learning how to use and hone this power we have to influence reality and literally manifest anything we want directly out of the field, from a new hip, to perhaps better eyesight, or a fit and healthy body, free of cancer, all the way to a new life.

But how is this done?

Healing Your Field, Healing Your Body

To heal, all that we need to do is purify our energy so that the energetic projection of our body is unobstructed. Then our atoms and molecules can align perfectly to this structure because there is no energetic interference to disrupt the image of our body as projected by our consciousness.

We do this by getting in the gap between our thoughts, where our beliefs no longer affect our reality, for, when we are not thinking, we are also free of beliefs and expectations. And by doing this we are aligning ourselves with universal principles, and matching our energy with the energies coming directly from the field of all-possibility—those high frequency energies of love, kindness, inspiration, passion, joy, and so on.

Your body is not the real you. Your body is merely a projection of what you believe yourself to be. If you could discover that you are pure consciousness, and that who you really are is an infinite creative awareness that is manifesting reality and co-creating reality with other aspects of yourself (because every being is an expression of the infinite universal consciousness we have labelled as God), *then you can start to take complete control over your body, your health, and your life.*

[A magnificent book to read in this field is *The Biology of Belief* by Bruce Lipton, and for a short introduction to it, you can visit ttps://www.youtube.com/watch?v=jjj0xVM4x1I]

Chronic pain, disease, illness, or the old injuries that you have in your body are not actually in your body, *they are in your mind.* More specifically, they are a function of your perception. Your atoms are always changing, and your molecules are too, but as new atoms come and as new molecules are formed, and your energetic field is telling them where to go, what to do, and how to align with one another.

Therefore, you are holding disease, illness, pain, and injuries within your consciousness, and thus, they are imprinted in your energetic field, and only then do they proceed to manifest in your physiology.

At that time, human beings will realize that the body is a manifestation of our highest self, and we can not only consciously manifest anything in life, but anything in *our bodies* as well. And one day we will reach a point where we can continually regenerate our bodies at will because we live from the field of infinite energy, and thus our bodies simply operate at a higher frequency so that we can live in them until our work is completed and we *choose* to move on.

But these changes are noticeable within the human body and mind even after a little bit of practice and training, so decide to feel and experience it for yourself, and learn how to meditate

[Louise Hay, in her book *Heal your Body*, says: 'In order to permanently eliminate a condition, we must first work to dissolve the mental cause.' She presents in this book a list of the causes of different types of diseases and the healing affirmations used to build new thought patterns that will produce health in mind and body.]

Our ability to heal is directly related to our level of attention and our level of belief. For example we can heal ourselves of any affliction, illness, disease, or injury that is possible so long as we have absolute certainty, a *knowing*, that we will be healed. This is directly achieved by accessing the most fundamental level of reality through deep meditation [or simply deeply believing in the Bible teachings, 'your faith has cured you'].

This is because at the fundamental level of reality, anything is possible, and the restructuring of reality is dictated entirely by our beliefs and expectations. We are pure energy, and there is infinite potential in that energy. It is entirely up to us what we choose to manifest out of the field in our lives and in our bodies.

You have no limitations, and nothing is impossible. It is only your beliefs which dictate what you can and cannot do'. (http://www.wakingtimes.com/2014/04/16/proof-human-body-projection-consciousness/ March, 2015).

As I said, you wish, and the universe will provide.

In this regard, Teal Swan says, 'Our emotions reflect our thoughts and the thoughts are vibrations. The vibrations keep us in a certain field of energy so we interact and attract people and situations with the same type of energy. The thoughts are creating emotions. The emotions are a biochemical feedback system which shows you at every moment of the day what your vibration is. If you feel sad, mean that you have low vibrational state; if you are happy, your frequency is high. It is up to us to choose to increase the positive vibration in our life. You get the positive vibration from all the things which make you to feel good and happy: music, places and people with high vibration like Nature, Water, Spiritual teachers, inspiring books, videos, movies, aromatherapy, doing physical exercise, doing random acts of kindness, etc. Everything that brings you joy is helping you to rise your frequency; the better you feel, the higher is your vibration and the quicker you will heal.'

To hear more about the ways of increasing your vibration/ frequency, go to http://www.youtube.com/watch?v=LB3ScXPViOM and *Ask Teal.*

> The more we can observe the reasons we put ourselves down, think negatively about ourselves or think there is something not loveable about ourselves, the more we can see what is blocking or stopping us from loving our true authentic self.

> Write it down if you have to. Take the time to sit quietly on your own and think of the reasons why you don't love yourself, feel self-conscious or think something isn't perfect about you.

> After you write down what do you think these things are, write down how you think each one got there. Did you see it in a movie? Learn it from friends, parents or other members of your family? Does society inoculate those thoughts in your mind this way?

> After you have gone through each one, go back and choose to first accept that you once thought of yourself that way. It's okay, at some point, we all have been through these things and it's often a normal part of personal development.

> Now realize how there is no real truth to the things you have mentioned about yourself as they are just perceptions created based on some false idea of who you think you are and what those things mean in terms

of love. The more you realize that you are not your appearance, career, hobbies and so forth, the more you begin to not rely on those things to love yourself.

Try looking at yourself in the mirror, look in your eyes and tell yourself you love yourself multiple times. See how this makes you feel. Is it easy? Awkward? Uncomfortable? Ask yourself why and reflect again on the answers that come up. The trick is the more you become aware of why you think these things about yourself, the more you realize they are stories and you begin to disempower them. From here it just takes continuing to disempower them as they creep back up as when you give them no truth and power, they dissipate because they are not true to begin with. They are just thought forms and ideas. (http://www.collective-evolution.com/2014/04/15/the-secret-to-feeling-loved-in-a-relationship-it-might-surprise-you/).

A powerful way to heal yourself and to eliminate the emotional cause of the disease is through forgiving others and yourself for past actions.

Barbara Brennan, in her book *Light Emerging*, teaches us how we can discover the roots of a disease and cure it through forgiveness. She gives us the following technique:

'Start writing a list of the things you must forgive yourself for.

Then, if you take each item and meditate on it for a few minutes several times a day and forgive yourself for it, you will lighten the burden on your heart. Forgiveness comes from the divine within. By praying for and experiencing your forgiveness, you connect with the divine within you. You become the divine within you.

The next questions are: How does each item that you forgive yourself for, show in your psyche and in your physical body? How does it show in your energy field? Trace it through all seven experiential levels of your field.

Where is the pain in your body that is associated with that unforgiving attitude that you have held toward yourself; and thereby maintained a negative connection with a particular individual that you find difficult to forgive? You see, healing always begins at home.

Within you, in the place an inch and a half to two inches above your navel, there is a beautiful star, the core star. It is the essence of your individuality. This essence is your divine individuality.

It is the centre of your being-ness. It is the centre of who you are in complete peace before, during, and beyond a lifetimes that you have ever experienced on your mother Earth.

Feel this place within you. You existed before this life.

You existed before all of the chaos and pain and strife that exists upon this earth, and you will continue to do so.

This centre of your being-ness is the centre of your divinity. From this place you are the centre of the entire Universe. It is from this place that you will heal. You will remember who you are, and you will help others remember who they are. For it is from the centre of your being that all of your actions arise. As soon as your actions become disconnected from the centre of your being, you are no longer aligned with your divine purpose.

Action disconnected from divine purpose creates pain and dis-ease. So, dear ones, centre yourselves into your core. It is from this centre that all forgiveness arises.

I should like you now to take the first item you found to forgive yourself for to your core.

Whatever it was that you created that needs forgiving was created in a manner that was disconnected from your center. As you moved to create, you disconnected from the center of your being' your actions became unaligned with your divine purpose and moved, perhaps ever so slightly, into shadow and forgetting. So if you take that which needs to be forgiven, bring it to the core star and simply hold it there, surround it and infuse it with love, you will, through this love, bring it back to the light. You will find your original purpose that arose from your center. Once having found this, you can move forth with the original creation. For in finding, surrounding, and infusing it with love and light, you will find forgiveness within yourself. I will give you a few moments now to bring forth self-forgiveness in this manner.

As this forgiveness streams through your being, you will find yourselves automatically forgiving others that may be involved in a particular situation that calls for forgiveness.

Feel a pillar of light within. Feel a star of light in your center, just above your navel. It is no accident that you are here. You have brought yourself to the very moment in your life, for your own purposes, which arise out of the deep and sacred longing that you carry above your heart. The more that you honour that longing, the more you will find yourself directly on your path in a life that is joyous and fulfilling, in a life that is creative and forgiving.

I would like you today to take one person with whom you are having difficulties in your life and begin working and praying to align yourself for forgiveness and healing. Healing requires forgiveness of both yourself and that individual. As you may know healing encompasses the entire life-indeed, all your lifetimes-and that which is beyond lifetimes. You exist in a realm much greater than the physical, which is defined by time and space. Time and space to you are only commodities of limitation that you have placed in this schoolroom, that you have created for your Self to learn within. You have created your Lesson, you have created your schoolroom, you have created your teachers within that schoolroom, and yet you are the master of all of this creation. You have come to this earth for your own purposes that are carried in your sacred longing.

Now I ask you, with regard to the person you have chosen, how have you betrayed your sacred longing and thereby created a situation in which self-forgiveness is needed? This may not be an easy answer that comes immediately. But if you focus on it and pray about it and connect it to your healing work, you will begin to understand.

Through your life experience, a deeper understanding of what is being said here will well up from the fountain of life within you. Yes, it is true that you create your experience of your life. It is of your design. You have designed it from the utmost wisdom within you. If there is pain then ask what that pain is saying to you, for pain arises out of forgetting who you are. Pain arises out of belief that the shadow reality is the true reality. The shadow reality is a result of forgetting who you are, which is based upon the belief that you are separate, or separated from God.

I tell you, dear ones, all disease, no matter what its form or manifestation, is the result of this forgetting. You have returned here, to this earth plane, to remember.

Do not be distressed by this.

Set your life-force in the direction of remembering, and its illumination will awaken the portions of your psyche that exist in shadow and in pain. When you illuminate them with the light of the divine, which exists within every cell of your body, within every cell of your being, the light shines into the shadow and the shadow begins to remember. Re-membering means to bring your members back together. Through illumination, you will re-member the portions of yourself and your body that have become dissociated and therefore dis-eased. It is a new beginning; yes, some pain is experienced, but it is a healing pain. The tears will wash your soul clear and clean, like fresh-fallen rain. Your cries will release what has been held for centuries, awaiting emergence. All of those blocks that have been talked about will flow and fill with life renewed. You will find yourself filled with much more energy. You will find your life moving into creativity and joy. You will find yourself being filled in a natural dance with all those around you, and with the universe.

But this requires forgiveness: forgiveness first of the self. What have you to forgive yourself for?'(*Light Emerging* by Barbara Brennan)

Maybe past 'wrong' decisions which changed your life, maybe some conflicts with family or friends which make you to feel guilty about your attitude, or just for not being good enough. Just tell yourself that, at that time and with that knowledge and state of mind, you have done your best.

All those past streams of guilt carried in your heart kept your soul in shadow and brought diseases to your body. Now it is time to release them and convince yourself that everything has happened as it should be. At that time and in that moment, you have done the best you could do, and there is no reason for you to feel guilty.

For a better understanding of those 'letting go' techniques, please read *Light Emerging* and *Hands of Light* by Barbara Brennan and *The Journey* by Brandon Bays.

Positive Emotions

'If someone wishes for good health, one must first ask oneself if he is ready to do away with the reasons for his illness. Only then is it possible to help him' (Hippocrates).

Definitely we can't cure any disease, especially cancer, if we live in fear of dying from it or if we repeat in our minds, 'This treatment doesn't work.' Our negative thoughts and emotions, as we discussed in the previous chapter, will determine our reality.

I know that it is very hard to stay positive when you are in pain or when the blood tests are worse than before, but this is the test set up for you to overcome your mind, your reality, and to create a different reality, the one which you like and are happy with.

> 'Humans experience an array of emotions, anything from happiness, to sadness to extreme joy and depression. Each one of these emotions creates a different feeling within the body. After all, our body releases different chemicals when we experience various things that make us happy and each chemical works to create a different environment within the body. For example if your brain releases serotonin, dopamine or oxytocin, you will feel good and happy. Convexly, if your body releases cortisol while you are stressed, you will have an entirely different feeling associated more with the body kicking into survival mode.

> What about when we are thinking negative thoughts all the time? Or how about when we are *thinking positive thoughts*? What about when we are not emotionally charged to neither positive nor negative? Let's explore how these affect our body and life'.(http://www. jewsnews.co.il/2014/10/14/shocking-the-effects-of-negative-thoughts-and-emotions-on-your-body/).

I noticed that all patients with cancer have an ongoing conflict with somebody: a family member, a friend, the government, the workplace, etc. The sad part of it is that they do not realize how much emphasis they put on this conflict and how much they are fuelling it, accumulating stress and negative energy which in the end feed the cancer. This conflict is amplified during a disease by the fear, discomfort, and pain, placing us in a vicious circle of stress and sickness and making us feel misunderstood, unloved, or neglected.

I was thinking that maybe the cancer produces certain chemicals to create nervousness and stress to maintain its acidic environment, which it likes so much (as it is able to form new blood vessels, angiogenesis, to feed itself). So maybe one way to get rid of it is to do whatever you can to be happy, positive, and optimistic. I know that it is hard when you are in pain and everybody around you is looking at you like you're almost a dead person, but it is a very important step in your healing to replace the conflict and sadness with happiness and peace!

Many around you will consider you crazy if you go dancing or go on trips or if you will search for a partner, but that is their business. Yours is to get healthy by using all methods and resources. This fight with cancer must be absolutely, not partially, because the cancer is aggressive and you nourished it for more than ten years before it appeared. Now you don't have so much time to eradicate it, so ignore others' opinions and do what you must.

> 'Usually, we spend a lot of time defining and judging what is to be considered as positive and what we consider to be as negative. The *brain* is a very powerful tool and as we define what something is or should be, we begin to have that result play out in our world. Have you ever noticed, for example that someone driving can get cut off and lose their lid, get angry and suddenly they are feeling negative, down and in bad mood? Whereas someone else can get cut off while driving and simply apply the break slightly and move on with their day as if nothing happened. In this case, the same experience yet one sees it as negative while the other doesn't. So are

things innately positive and negative? Or do we define things as positive and negative?

After thinking about it for a moment you might realize that there are in fact no positive or negative experiences other than what we define as such and the way how we react to them. Therefore our very perception of an experience or situation has the ultimate power on how we feel when it's happening and how our bodies will be affected. While we can always work to move beyond our definitions of each experience and move into a state of mind/awareness/consciousness where we simply accept each experience for what it is and use it as a learning grounds for us.

The *connection between your mind and body* is very powerful and although it cannot be visually seen, the effects on your physical body are profound. We can have an overall positive mental attitude and deal directly with our internal challenges and in turn create a healthy lifestyle or we can be in negative, have self destructive thoughts and not deal with our internal issues.

Our emotions and experiences are mostly energy and they can be stored in the cellular memory of our bodies. Have you ever experienced something in your life that left an emotional mark or pain in a certain area of your body? Almost as if you can still feel something that may have happened to you? It is likely because in that area of your body you still hold energy released from that experience that is remaining in that area. [Sometimes before exams, I would feel like a knot or like a heavy stone is in my stomach.]

When you have a pain, tightness or injuries in certain areas, it's often related to something emotionally you are feeling within yourself. At first glance it may not seem this way because we are usually very out of touch with ourselves and our emotions in this fast paced world, but it's often the truth. When I've had chronic pains in my back, knees, neck or shoulders, it wasn't exercise, physio or anything in a physical sense that healed it, it was when I dealt with the emotions behind it. I know this because I spent the time and money going to physio and even though I wanted and believed I would get better, something wasn't being addressed still. The more I addressed the unconscious thought pattern and emotions throughout my body, the more things loosened up and pain went away.

[Talk with your body and ask, 'What is the root of this pain? What is the emotional charge of it? What was the event or experience which provoked it?' A real help in practicing this technique is Dr Hawkins's book *Healing and Recovery* and *The Journey* by Brandon Bays.]

When you get sick or are feeling a lot of tightness and pain, often your body is asking you to observe yourself and find peace once again within yourself and your environment. It's all a learning and growing process we don't have to judge nor fear.' (http://www.jewsnews. co.il/2014/10/14/shocking-the-effects-of-negative-thoughts-and-emotions-on-your-body/)

Davis Suzuki wrote in 'The Sacred Balance': 'Condensed molecules from breath exhaled from verbal expressions of anger, hatred, and jealousy, contain toxins. Accumulated over 1 hr, these toxins are enough to kill 80 guinea pigs!' Can you now imagine the harm you are doing to your body when you stay within negative emotions or unprocessed emotional experience throughout the body?'

'Remember, you have all the power in you to get through anything life throws at you. Instead of labelling with perception the concepts of negative and positive as it relates to each experience you have in your life, try to see things from a big picture standpoint. Ask yourself, how can this help me to see or learn something? Can I use this to shift my perception or clear some emotion within myself? Realize something within another and accept it? Whatever it may be, instead of simply reacting, slow things down and observe. You will find you have the tools to process emotions and illness quickly when you see them for what they are and explore why they came up. If you believe you will get sick all the time, and believe you have pain because it's all out of your control, you will continue to have it all in an uncontrollable manner until you realize the control you have over much of what we attract within the body.' (http://www.jewsnews.co.il/2014/10/14/shocking-the-effects-of-negative-thoughts-and-emotions-on-your-body/ December 2014)

'Emotions coordinate our behaviour and physiological states during survival-salient events and pleasurable interactions. Even though we are often consciously aware of our current emotional state, such as anger or happiness, the mechanisms giving rise to these subjective sensations have remained unresolved. Here we used a topographical self-report tool to reveal that different emotional states are associated with topographically distinct and culturally universal bodily sensations; these sensations could underlie our conscious emotional experiences. Monitoring the topography of emotion-triggered bodily sensations brings forth a unique tool for emotion research and could even provide a biomarker for emotional disorders' (http://themindunleashed.org/2014/01/research-mapping-human-emotions-shows-strong-mind-body-connection.html, December 2014).

I came across an interesting chart that shows the connection between our emotions and the pain manifested in different areas of our body. It is called Emotional Pain Chart: The Mental Thought Patterns That Form Our Experiences, and you can see it at http://www.jewsnews. co.il/2014/10/14/shocking-the-effects-of-negative-thoughts-and-emotions-on-your-body/.

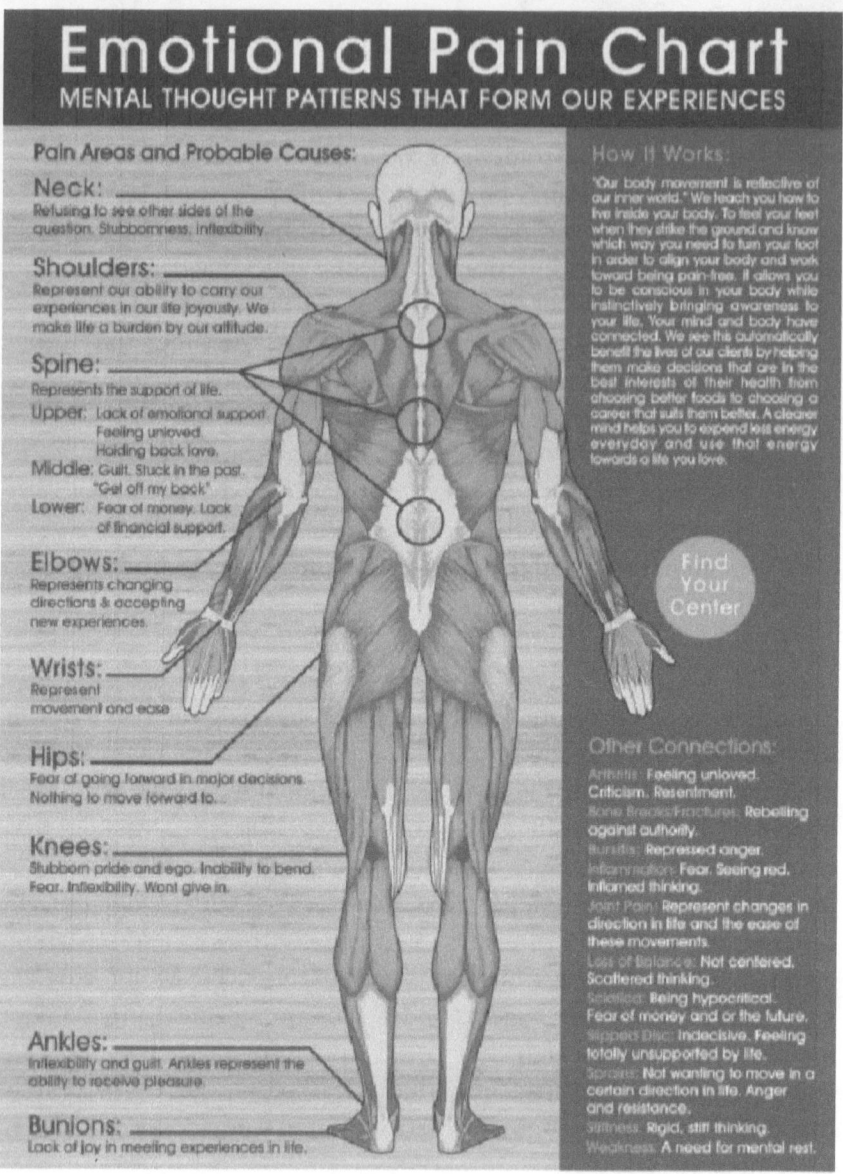

Emotional Pain Chart
MENTAL THOUGHT PATTERNS THAT FORM OUR EXPERIENCES

Pain Areas and Probable Causes:

Neck:
Refusing to see other sides of the question. Stubbornness, inflexibility.

Shoulders:
Represent our ability to carry our experiences in our life joyously. We make life a burden by our attitude.

Spine:
Represents the support of life.
Upper: Lack of emotional support.
Feeling unloved.
Holding back love.
Middle: Guilt. Stuck in the past.
"Get off my back"
Lower: Fear of money. Lack of financial support.

Elbows:
Represents changing directions & accepting new experiences.

Wrists:
Represent movement and ease

Hips:
Fear of going forward in major decisions. Nothing to move forward to.

Knees:
Stubborn pride and ego. Inability to bend. Fear. Inflexibility. Won't give in.

Ankles:
Inflexibility and guilt. Ankles represent the ability to receive pleasure.

Bunions:
Lack of joy in meeting experiences in life.

How It Works:
"Our body movement is reflective of our inner world." We teach you how to live inside your body. To feel your feet when they strike the ground and know which way you need to turn your foot in order to align your body and work toward being pain-free. It allows you to be conscious in your body while instinctively bringing awareness to your life. Your mind and body have connected. We see this automatically benefit the lives of our clients by helping them make decisions that are in the best interests of their health from choosing better foods to choosing a career that suits them better. A clearer mind helps you to expend less energy everyday and use that energy towards a life you love.

Find Your Center

Other Connections:
Arthritis: Feeling unloved. Criticism. Resentment.
Bone Breaks/Fractures: Rebelling against authority.
Bursitis: Repressed anger.
Inflammation: Fear. Seeing red. Inflamed thinking.
Joint Pain: Represent changes in direction in life and the ease of these movements.
Loss of Balance: Not centered. Scattered thinking.
Sciatica: Being hypocritical. Fear of money and or the future.
Slipped Disc: Indecisive. Feeling totally unsupported by life.
Sprains: Not wanting to move in a certain direction in life. Anger and resistance.
Stiffness: Rigid, stiff thinking.
Weakness: A need for mental rest.

'A team of scientists in Finland has used a topographical self-reported method to reveal the effects that different emotional states have on bodily sensations. After five experiments and over 700 participants from Finland, Sweden and Taiwan, who reported where on their bodies they felt different emotions, the scientists discovered surprising consistencies. Their research findings were published in the *Proceedings*

of the National Academy of Sciences.' (http://themindunleashed.
org/2014/01/research-mapping-human-emotions-shows-strong-mind-
body-connection.html).

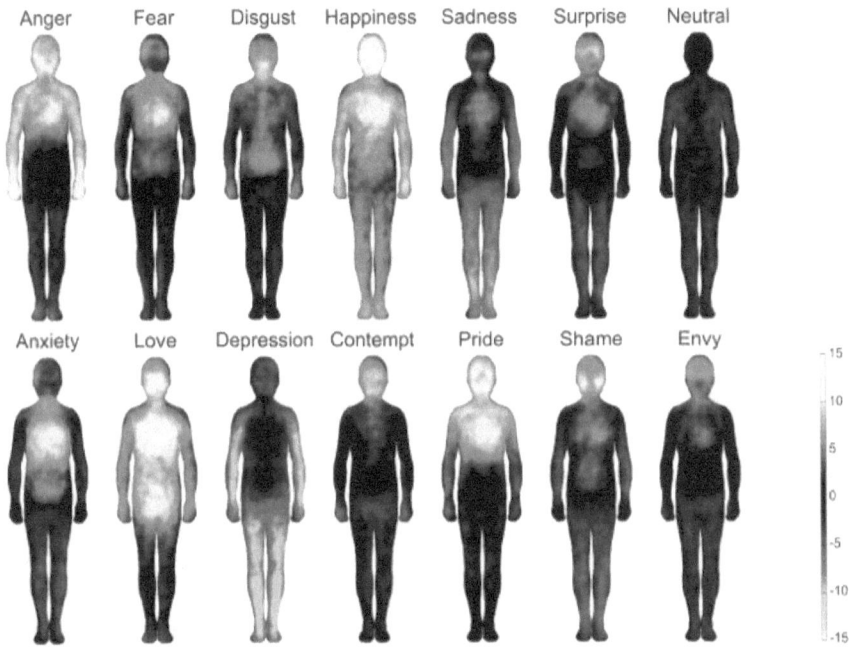

Image source: Lauri Nummenmaa et al. (http://www.pnas.
org/content/early/2013/12/26/1321664111.full.pdf).

They concluded: 'Most basic emotions were associated with sensations
of elevated activity in the upper chest area, likely corresponding to
changes in breathing and heart rate. Similarly, sensations in the head area
were shared across all emotions, reflecting probably both physiological
changes in the facial area (i.e., facial musculature activation, skin
temperature, lacrimation) as well as the felt changes in the contents
of mind triggered by the emotional events. Sensations in the upper
limbs were most prominent in approach-oriented emotions, anger and
happiness, whereas sensations of decreased limb activity were a defining
feature of sadness. Sensations in the digestive system and around the
throat region were mainly found in disgust. In contrast with all of the

other emotions, happiness was associated with enhanced sensations all over the body.'

'Emotional feelings are associated with discrete, yet partially overlapping maps of bodily sensations, which could be at the core of the emotional experience. These results thus support models assuming that somatosensation and embodiment play critical roles in emotional processing. Unravelling the subjective bodily sensations associated with human emotions may help us to better understand mood disorders such as depression and anxiety, which are accompanied by altered emotional processing), and somatosensation. Topographical changes in emotion-triggered sensations in the body could thus provide a novel biomarker for emotional disorders.' (http://www.pnas.org/content/early/2013/12/26/1321664111.full.pdf March 2015).

'This research is another great example of the mind and body connection. Our brain sends signals to the body as we deal with certain situations, causing certain physiological changes without any thought on our part. These bodily sensations in turn could be helping the mind to consciously recognize what emotions we are having. This type of research could help explain why making an effort to smile more or avoid negative thoughts and words, can alter our brain, improve our mood, and change our general disposition [and even the body structure].' (http://www.wakingtimes.com/2014/01/03/research-mapping-human-emotions-shows-strong-mind-body-connection/).

'The best way to overcome undesirable or negative thoughts and feelings is to cultivate the positive ones.' says William Atkinson.

The article 'The Effect of Positive Emotions on Our Health' (found at http://fractalenlightenment.com/27015/life/the-effect-of-positive-emotions-on-our-health) says:

> "It is important we recognise our thoughts and emotions and be aware of their effect not only on our health but also our relationships and our surroundings. Positive emotions makes you feel happy and joyful. Everything

around you seems beautiful, you enjoy the moment and things seem to fall into place.

Barbara Fredrickson, one of the long-time researchers and author on positive emotions, has shown how cultivating positivity can transform us at a cellular level and actually shape who we are.

Fredrickson's theory of positive emotions, 'Broaden-and-build' suggests that positive emotions lead to novel, expansive behaviour, and these actions, over time, lead to lasting emotional resilience, flourishing and meaningful social relationships.

Positive emotions or behaviour—like playfulness, gratitude, awe, love, interest, serenity, and feeling of interconnectedness to others—broadens our perspective, opens our mind and heart as we feel completely in tune with our environment. Like the flowers that open up when the sun rises, the same way positive emotions bring light and joy back in our lives.

According to Fredrickson, 'Negative emotions are necessary for us to flourish, and positive emotions are by nature subtle and fleeting; the secret is not to deny their transience but to find ways to increase their quantity.' Rather than trying to eliminate negativity, she recommends we balance negative feelings with positive ones.

Lets see the physical and emotional benefits of positive emotions :

- Positive emotions have been shown to benefit individuals with cardiovascular disease.
- Lower blood pressure and risk for cardiovascular disease
- Better sleep, fewer colds, headaches, aches and pain, and a greater sense of overall happiness

- Expands our perception of what lies in our peripheral vision
- Research suggests that even more abstract positive emotions like hope and curiosity offer protective benefits from diseases like high blood pressure and diabetes.
- Studies show that positive emotions help a person to overcome negative emotions faster and be more resilient and be able to cope with a difficult situation.
- People are more playful when happy, so that leads better physical fitness, regular exercise or increased flexibility. (so its important to engage in an activity that makes you happy)
- People who experience warmer, more upbeat emotions may have better physical health because they make more social connections

When you delve in that happy space, more possibilities and new ideas emerge and our creativity flows. Happiness and joy transform us, although you might not stay in that state all the time. There will be days when you feel down and out, but if we observe our emotions and divert our mind and think of the happy moments, you will find the negative emotion fading away.

Don't forget negative, repressed emotions can have detrimental effect on our body, mind and spirit. It takes control over you and makes you feel down, gloomy, unhealthy and it's an unpleasant state to be in [which, slowly, if you don't overcome it, will become a habit].

Nothing like a good humour to drive the negativity away, works for me. So increase your daily diet of positivity or engage in activities that bring about happy feelings either meditation, exercise, yoga, laughter clubs, walk, music, painting, and so on. Love your life and yourself.

Positive feelings also help us live in the present moment and believe in oneness and interconnectedness with everything around us.' (http://fractalenlightenment.com/27015/life/the-effect-of-positive-emotions-on-our-health)

For more info, go to:

'Exploring the Nature of Mind and Our Holographic Brain' from http://www.projectglobalawakening.com/2014/03/29/nature-of-mind/

http://themindunleashed.org/2014/04/proof-human-body-projection-consciousness.html.

Meditation/Hypnosis

Another useful treatment for cancer which you may consider is hypnotherapy.

I had a few amazing sessions of regressive hypnosis with my nephew Vlad, who is a successful hypnotherapist in Romania (see the chapter 5)

Hypnosis is the creation of a relaxed state of being in which the mind stops multitasking and begins to focus on one particular point.

> Hypnotherapy is the treatment of a variety of health conditions by hypnotism or by inducing prolonged sleep.

> Hypnotherapy is thought to date back to the healing practices of ancient Greece and Egypt. Many religions such as Judaism, Christianity, Islam, and others have attributed trance-like behavior to spiritual or divine possession.

> Austrian physician, Franz Mesmer (1734–1815), is credited with being the first person to scientifically investigate the idea of hypnotherapy, in 1779, to treat a

variety of health conditions. Mesmer studied medicine at the University of Vienna and received his medical degree in1766. Mesmer is believed to have been the first doctor to understand the relationship of psychological trauma to illness'.(http://medical-dictionary.thefreedictionary. com/hypnotherapy

To treat nervous disorders, he induced a trance like state in his patients (mesmerism), and these techniques became the foundation for modern-day hypnotherapy.

He later became interested in the healing effects of magnetism on the human body, believing that each body contains fluid with magnetic properties, which can influence the well-being of the person.

In his healing techniques, Mesmer used his hands to transmit magnetic waves over the sick body with the idea of influencing the flow of the magnetic fluid.

Though Mesmer's technique appeared to be quite successful in the treatment of his patients, he was the subject of scorn and ridicule from the medical comunity and a very distinguished panel of investigators, including Benjamin Franklin, the French chemist Antoine Laurent Lavoisier, and physician Jacques Guillotin, was convened to investigate him. Even they acknowledged that the patients presented noticeable improvements, but the method used was classified as quackery.

It took more than two hundred years for hypnotherapy to become incorporated into medical treatment. In 1955, the British Medical Association approved the use of hypnotherapy as a valid medical treatment, with the American Medical Association (AMA) giving its approval in 1958.

Hypnotherapy involves achieving a psychological state of awareness that is different from the ordinary state of consciousness. While in a hypnotic state, a variety of phenomena can occur including alterations in memory, receptivity to suggestion, paralysis, sweating, and blushing. All of these changes can be produced or removed in the hypnotic state. Many studies have shown that roughly 90% of the population is capable of being hypnotized.

This state of awareness can be achieved by relaxing the body, focusing on breathing, and shifting attention away from the external environment.

Hypnotherapy is the treatment of a variety of health conditions by hypnotism or by inducing prolonged sleep.

Pioneers in this field, such as James Braid and James Esdaile discovered that hypnosis could be used to successfully anesthetize patients for surgeries. James Braid accidentally discovered that one of his patients began to enter a hypnotic state while staring at a fixed light as he waited for his eye examination to begin.

[Braid changed the term *mesmerism* into term *hypnotism*, derived from the Greek word for *sleep*.] Around 1900, there were very few preoperative anesthetic drugs available. Patients were naturally apprehensive when facing surgery. One out of four hundred patients would die, not from the surgical procedure, but from the anesthesia.

Dr. Henry Munro was one of the first physicians to use hypnotherapy to alleviate patient fear of surgery. He would get his patients into a hypnotic state and discuss their fear with them, telling that they would feel a lot better following surgery.

Ether was the most common anesthetic at that time, and Dr. Munro found that he was able to perform surgery using only about 10% of the usual amount of ether.

Research on the effectiveness of hypnotherapy on a variety of medical conditions is extensive. In one study, the use of hypnotherapy did not seem to alter the core symptoms in the treatment of attention deficit hyperactivity disorder (ADHD), but was useful in managing the associated symptoms [like tics, sleep disorders, and other disturbances].

Hypnotherapy is being studied in children who have common, chronic problems and to aid in relieving pain. Children are particularly good candidates for hypnotherapy because their lack of worldly experience enables them to move easily between the rational world and their imagination. Studies with children have shown responses to hypnotherapy ranging from diminished pain and anxiety during a number of medical procedures, a 50% range in reduction of symptoms or a complete resolution of a medical condition, and a reduction in use of anti-nausea medication and vomiting during chemotherapy for childhood cancers.

The use of hypnotherapy with cancer patients is another area being investigated. A meta-analysis of 116 studies showed very positive results of using hypnotherapy with cancer patients. Ninety-two percent showed a positive effect on depression; 93% showed a positive effect on physical wellbeing; 81% showed a positive effect on vomiting; and 92% showed a positive effect on pain.' (thttp://medical-dictionary.thefreedictionary. com/hypnotherapy)

Now, let's make a summary of the all the natural therapies to have a whole picture of them.

CHAPTER 4

ALTERNATIVE CANCER THERAPIES

There are many alternative cancer therapies available. The following list contains the one which are used the most. Before you start on any new treatment, make sure that you have all the correct information about that product/drug, and I suggest that you consult two to three naturopaths or GPs to hear their opinions on the effectiveness of the treatment and its side effects. The therapies presented below are just for your information, and you need to do research about them before you start the treatment. Also keep in mind that in every week there are new discoveries and new trials to validate alternative therapies, so stay informed.

I classified the most important therapies into four groups: nutritional therapy, environmental therapy, electronic therapy, and drugs/chemical therapy.

1. The Nutritional Therapy

Many centres are using a variety of food therapies to treat cancer. The most important are:

a) Diet Therapy

- Gerson's Therapy was developed by Dr Max Gerson in 1950 and consists of daily eating vegetable soups, drinking up to fifteen glasses of juice, and taking supplements, such as iodine, potassium, vitamin B12, Lugol's solution, and pancreatic enzymes. Coffee enemas will clean and eliminate the toxins in the blood, as caffeine is rapidly absorbed through the lower bowel to the liver stimulating its function.
- Budwig diet/flaxseed oil therapy was introduced in 1930 by Dr Johanna Budwig, a German pharmacologist, physicist, and seven-time Nobel Prize nominee. She discovered that without the proper metabolism of fats in our bodies, every vital function and every organ is affected. She combined flaxseed oil, which contains unsaturated fats, and cottage cheese, which is rich in sulfur protein (read more at http://www.cancertutor.com/budwig/).
- Hippocrates diet developed by Ann Wigmore allows the body to correct its problems and heal naturally through a diet of fresh fruits, vegetables, grains, nuts, and super-nutritious foods, such as sprouts and wheatgrass juice, most of them prepared without cooking.
- Macrobiotic diet is generally vegetarian and consists largely of whole grains, cereals, and cooked vegetables carefully selected to balance the yin and yang energies in the body. Based on Asian traditions, those two energies need to be in balance in order to achieve health and well-being.

b) Herbal/Plant Therapy

The most used herbs and plants are:

- Cannabinoids from cannabis are a group of compounds that include cannabinol and other active constituents of cannabis. They activate cannabinoid receptors in the body. The body itself produces substances called endocannabinoids, which play an important role in many processes within the body, including the immune response. See chapter 1.

- Artemesia, also known as wormwood, is a safe, non-toxic, and inexpensive treatment for cancer used mostly in Chinese medicine.
- Mistletoe extract (Iscador) stimulates the body's immune response to infection and diseases and induces cancer cell death through apoptosis.
- Essiac tea is an herbal mixture composed of slippery elm, burdock, Indian rhubarb, sorrel, and other ingredients. It was named after a nurse in Canada, Rene Caisse (*Essiac* is *Caisse* spelled backwards). Caisse gave the formula to a company in Canada who markets the product today. Indian rhubarb contains benzaldehyde, one of the components of vitamin B17 (laetrile).
- Graviola or soursop (*Annona muricata*) is a tree growing in the rainforests of the Amazon, Australia, and Fiji. Research shows that the extracts from graviola leaves and bark inhibit the herpes simplex virus and have antiviral, anti-parasitic, anti-rheumatic, and cytoxic effects, especially on prostate, colon, and pancreatic cancer. For more information, go to http://www.graviola.org.
- Hoxsey is an herbal concoction used first in 1924 by Harry M. Hoxsey. It is composed of barberry root, buckthorn bark, poke root, blood root, burdock root, and stillinga root. It is administered in two forms: orally or topically (through an ointment if the tumour is close to the surface of the skin). Hoxey's grandfather created the formula after observing his horses curing themselves of cancer by eating certain plants.
- Pau d'Arco is a tree growing in South America. The bark extract contains lapachol and twenty other compounds that have great results in treating cancer, lupus erythematosus, parasitosis, and diabetes.
- Radium weed, also known as petty spurge or *Euphorbia peplus*, has been used as a treatment for skin problems for hundreds of years, especially to treat warts and some types of skin cancer.
- Red clover contains (according to the American National Cancer Institute) four anti-tumour compounds.
- Cat's claw is to not be confused with the red clover. Cat's claw is a rich source of phytochemicals. It has more than thirty known constituents, including at least seventeen alkaloids, along with glycosides, tannins, flavonoids, sterol fractions, and other compounds.

- Herb Robert (*Geranium robertianum*) is known also as Herb robertianum, St Robert, storkbill, cranesbill, red robin, fox geranium, St Robert's Wort, bloodwort, felonwort, dragon's blood. Herb Robert is an enigmatic herb that has a miraculous effect in some forms of cancer and boosts the immune system.
- Saw palmetto is often used in the treatment of prostate cancer.
- Mushrooms: *maitake*, shiitake, cordyceps, reishi, coriolus, *Phellinus linteus*, *Agaricus*, and others.
- Aloe vera helps the body fight infections and malignant cells by improving the immune system and acting as a detoxifier. You can use the plant as it is, or you can buy it in pill form, called Ambrotose, or as a drink from health shops.
- Haelan is a promising nutritional-based anticancer agent made from liquid soybean extract. Its array of benefits include blocking of cancer cell's blood supplies and enzymatic activity, tumour reduction, and boosting of the immune system. It has also been found to help relieve the side effects of conventional cancer therapies.
- There are many other plants known by the native people of remote villages which can be studied and used in the future.

c) <u>Vitamins-and-Minerals Therapy</u>

Vitamins-and-minerals therapy involves a combination of acid-neutralizing minerals—like calcium, magnesium, bicarbonate soda, potassium, rubidium, and especially caesium—and a healthy vegetarian diet to supply proper mineralization and to correct the acid–alkaline balance of the body by alkalinizing the cancer cells (neutralize their acid nature), as the cancer cells do not survive in higher pH.

The most used vitamins and minerals are: Percy's powder, magnesium, calcium, potassium, zinc, vitamin B17 (laetrile), vitamin B12, vitamin C, vitamin D3, CoQ 10 enzymes, amino acids (we discussed all in the previous chapter).

Poly-MVA is a powerful antioxidant supplement composed of polynucleotide reductase plus minerals, vitamins, and amino acids.

d) Metabolic Therapy

'Metabolic therapy is based on the belief that toxic substances in food and the environment build up in the body and create chemical imbalances that lead to diseases such as cancer, arthritis, and multiple sclerosis. Metabolic therapy uses a combination of special diets, enzymes, nutritional supplements, and other measures in an attempt to remove 'toxins' from the body and strengthen the body's defences against disease.' (http://health-axis.com/tony-pantalleresco-radio-show-notes-week-ending-18th-of-august-2013/).

Dr Kelly and Dr Nicholas Gonzales are well known for their use of metabolic therapy in treating cancer. Dr Kelly's book is online at www. drkelley.com/CANLIVER55.html.

2. Environmental Therapies

The second group of therapies I call environmental therapies because they contain therapies which help us in connection with our environment.

a) Oxygen/Ozone Therapy

This therapy introduces high concentrations of oxygen into the body, using pressure chambers, chemical compounds, liquid oxygen, ozone treatment, etc. Using the theory that cancer cells do not live in a healthy, oxygenated environment, Nobel Prize winner Dr Otto Warburg showed that treating tumoural cells with oxygen may stop their growth or even help to return them to normal.

- Hydrogen peroxide is administered intravenously and supplies an abundance of oxygen to the cancer site.
- Hyperbaric oxygen therapy is mostly used for strokes and brain damage, but it has been used by some American clinics for treating cancer.
- Ozone (O_3) therapy has been used in Europe for many years, as it has powerful antiviral and antibacterial properties. In the body, ozone creates an oxygen-rich environment that may force

cancer cells to shift from an anaerobic metabolism to a normal function.

b) Hyperthermia

Hyperthermia is used mostly for tumours located near the surface of the body by increasing the temperature for one hour or so. By increasing the temperature of the body, it also increases the blood circulation and the oxygen supply to the tissue, causing the death of the malignant cells. In Melbourne you can have hyperthermia treatments at NIIM in Hawthorn.

c) Hydrotherapy/Sauna

'Under the general heading of hydrotherapy, there are several techniques. These include baths and showers, neutral baths, sitz baths, contrast sitz baths, foot baths, cold mitten friction rub, steam inhalation, sauna, hot compresses, cold compresses, alternating hot and cold compresses, heating compresses, body wrap, wet sheet pack, and salt glow.'(http://www.naturaltherapypages.com.au/article/hydrotherapy).

Hydrotherapy treatments increase:

- heart rate and respiratory rate
- increase metabolism, which is important for healing
- increased perspiration, which assists in detoxification.

Read more at:

http://www.naturaltherapypages.com.au/article/hydrotherapy#ixzz393HsijcL

http://www.treating-cancer-alternatively.com/Hydrotherapy.html.

d) Meditation, Massage, Aromatherapy

Over the last twenty years, clinical trials have studied meditation as a way of reducing stress in both the mind and body. Most of the recent research has focused on mindfulness based stress reduction. The trials have shown that meditation can help to reduce anxiety, tiredness, stress, chronic pain and sleep problems. It can also help to lower blood pressure.

Some scientific evidence shows that meditation can help to relieve particular symptoms and improve quality of life for people with cancer. Research has shown that it can

- Improve your mood
- Improve your ability to concentrate
- Reduce severe depression (studies have looked at mindfulness based stress reduction)
- Boost the immune system. (http://www.cancerresearchuk.org/)

3. Electronic Therapies

a)   Electrotherapy (Galvanotherapy or Electro-Cancer Treatment (ECT))

This was developed in Europe by Dr Björn Nordenström and Dr Rudolf Pekar. The technique is using a positively-charged platinum, gold, or silver needle placed in the tumour and other negatively-charged needles around the tumour. ECT works by using voltages of 6 to 15 volts, depending on tumour size, influencing the acid/alkaline (pH) levels within the tumour and causing electrolysis of its tissue, which is more susceptible to direct current than the normal tissue.

b)   Magnetic Resonance or Bio-Resonance

Bio-resonance therapy was invented in Germany in 1977 by Franz Morell and his son-in-law, Erich Rasche, an engineer. The technique uses a device to create a change of 'bio-resonance' in cells, and this reverses the change caused by the disease. The device isolates and pinpoints pathogens' responses from the mixture of responses it receives via the electrodes. Practitioners claim that transmitting these transformed signals over the same electrodes can generate healing signals that have the curative effect.

This category includes *rife machines*, *zappers*, and Metatron, a device which I tried myself (thanks to a kind osteopath from NIIM, Dr Simon Armstrong).

'Metatron is a **revolutionary computer-non-linear scanner** that provides accurate diagnosis of any energetic disturbance within the person. Once the Metatron locates energetic disturbance, it continues to seek for the root cause of the disrupted energy flow—to cellular level and even to chromosomes and gene level also.' (http://metatherapy.com. au/f-a-q-about-metatron-metatherapy-and-health/).

'Every organ has an electromagnetic code and the computer will analyse each one of them on automatic or manual mode. The Metatron will establish a health card allowing to correct electromagnetic imbalances and recommends naturopathic treatments.' (http://www.nlsdiag.com/).

'After completing the analysis, Metatron Non Linear Scanner stimulates body's healing process by using Metatherapy (sometimes referred to as 'Meta-Therapy'). In effect Metatherapy is stimulating the target area with appropriate resonate frequencies, in fact re-energizing the targeted are whether cells or organ. The Metatron scanner records the condition of the treatments and allows the practitioner to compare the before and after changes. This way the Metatron makes it easy for the practitioner and 'patient' to be well informed about the progress and effectiveness of the therapy.'(http://metatherapy.com. au/f-a-q-about-metatron-metatherapy-and-health/).

In Australia I know a Metatrone distributor in Queensland (www. kalayaproducts.com.au). Be aware that some of those ultrasound/ magnetic therapies may have negative side effects. As an example, using Radachlorine with sonodynamic therapy in bone treatment can 'bleach' the bones, making them brittle and prone to fractures. Do research, and find testimonies before you use any of those techniques.

One of the pioneers in the use of zappers and anti-parasitic herbals is Dr Clark. Her website is www.drclark.net.

For more info, search:

www.kalayaproducts.com.au

http://www.nlsdiag.com/

http://metatherapy.com.au/f-a-q-about-metatron-metatherapy-and-health/.

4. The Drugs Therapy

a)   Antineoplastons

Antineoplastons are amino acid compounds discovered in 1967 that are present in the blood and urine of healthy people but are deficient in cancer patients.

b)   Cancell/Protocel

Cancell/Protocel is a compound discovered in 1935 which can lower the energy of the body, starving the cancer cells, which are great consumers of energy. The technique had a success of 70–80 per cent, but the FDA didn't approve the mass production. It is now being used occasionally as many other cancer treatments.

c) Hydrazine Sulfat

Hydrazine sulfat is a chemical that inhibits the liver's production of sugar, starving the cancer cells. You can find more information on this at Syracuse Cancer Research Institute's website at http://scri.ngen.com/ or http://www.kathykeeton-cancer.com/.

d) 714X (Naessen) or Immunostim

714X is a combination of ammonium, camphor, phosphors, and silicate acting based on the microorganism theory of cancer.

e) Insulin Potentiation Therapy (IPT)

'The insulin works on the malignant cell membranes and allows chemotherapy to target them. Thus, it is the chemotherapy that kills the cancer cells, however, because of the insulin, the amount of chemotherapy needed is greatly reduced. Thus, the chemotherapy is much more potent, much less chemotherapy is needed, and far less side-effects are experienced.' (http://www.cancertutor.com/ipt/).

f) Controlled Amino Acid Treatment (CAAT)

'There are 20 standard amino acids (as well as many non-standard ones) of which 9 or 10 are considered to be '**essential amino acids**.' The essential amino acids cannot be made inside the human body, and have to be ingested through food. Occasionally an amino acid can become 'conditionally essential' to help our bodies. A growing tumour needs, more so than any normal tissue, a good supply of blood to thrive. Normal cells have an integral blood supply, while cancer cells must create new blood vessels as it grows. Elastin is a protein essential to the formation of new blood vessels, therefore cancers must be deprived of elastin to minimise or inhibit growth. The constituent amino acids found in elastin are: proline, leucine, isoleucine, valine and glycine; the latter comprising almost one quarter of the make-up of the elastin'. (http://aminoacidstudies.org/cancer/, December 2014).

g)   Alpha Lipoic Acid

Alpha lipolic acid is present in almost all foods, but slightly more so in the kidney, heart, liver, spinach, broccoli, and yeast extract. It is an organosulphur compound with antioxidant effect and role in cell division.

h)   Chelation Therapy

> Chelation therapy refers to the injection or consumption of chelating agents for the purpose of eliminating from the body undesirable substances such as heavy metals, chemical toxins, mineral deposits, and fatty plaques. For example, in the arteries, the chelation agent binds to the calcium in plaques.
>
> The most widely used and studied chelating agent is EDTA (Ethylene Diamine Tetraacetic Acid), which is a synthetic amino acid. Where amino acids are the building blocks of protein.
>
> A Swiss study published in 1980 by Drs. Blumer W., Reich T., reported 90% fewer cancer deaths and 86% less cardiovascular events during an 18 year follow-up period in patients who took a series of 20 preventive chelation treatments.
>
> (http://www.issels.com/newissels/treatment-summary/chelation/).

There are a few ways to administrate chelation:

- chelation with calcium disodium EDTA
- chelation with magnesium EDTA in the form of intravenous injections
- oral EDTA in the form of capsules
- EDTA suppositories.

See more at
http://www.issels.com/treatment/chelation.aspx#sthash.Pe6xSUuT.dpuf.

i)   Interferon

Interferon, or the Koch serum, stimulates the growth of certain disease-fighting blood cells in the immune system, and it helps slow tumour growth.

j)   Interleukin-2

It is a protein that regulates the activities of white blood cells, which are responsible for immunity. IL-2 is part of the body's natural response to microbial infection. Recent studies show that a combination of interleukin and melatonin is very efficient in the lung cancer treatment.

k)   Enzymatic Therapy

Enzymes are natural proteins that stimulate and accelerate biological reactions in the body. Digestive enzymes, many of which are made in the pancreas, break down food and help with the absorption of nutrients into the blood. Metabolic enzymes build new cells; repair damaged ones in the blood, tissues, and organs; and can dissolve the protein coat of the cancerous cells, making them more accessible to the body's defence system. In Europe, the most used enzyme is Wobe-Mugos, which is approved by FDA as an orphan drug. More information about this therapy can be found in the book *World without Cancer* by Edward Griffin.

l)   GcMAF Protein Treatment

> GcMAF is a human protein which in a healthy person, has 11 actions discovered so far, including two on cells, three excellent effects on the brain, and 6 on cancer. Amongst these it acts as a 'director' of your immune system. But viruses and malignant cells like cancer send out an enzyme called Nagalase that prevents production of your GcMAF and neutralises your immune system. So diseases become chronic, and cancer cells grow unchecked.

Minutes after a receiving a dose, 10 of the actions restart. In three weeks of two GcMAF 0.25ml doses a week, your immune system is rebuilt to above normal strength. You need two doses a week for typically 24 weeks for many diseases and early cancers, up to seven (one ml)doses a week and a year for stage 4 cancers. The disease is then taken down without side effects, and successfully in up to 80% of cases. (.https://gcmaf.se/ gcmaf-science/how-gcmaf-works/).

m) Vaccines

The aim of cancer vaccines is to help the body's immune system to recognize and destroy the malignant cells. The most used vaccines are:

Dendritic cell cancer vaccines: 'Dendritic cells (DCs) represent unique antigen-producing cells capable of sensitizing T cell. Inoculation with new dendritic cells alerts the immune system to the presence of cancer and restarts proper immune function. This serves to mobilize the power of the immune system to identify cancer and combat it. These dendritic cells are cultured from the patient's own white blood cells (so they are described as 'autologous'). Initially, after a simple blood draw, the blood is sent to a high-tech medical laboratory where specially trained cell biologists and technicians separate out certain white blood cells (monocytes) from the blood. These cells are then cultured and transformed in seven days into a new generation dendritic cells. This new generation of vital, activated dendritic cells is re-introduced into the patient's body through simple injections' (http://prsync.com/ leading-edge-medical-ltd/lemed-adding-immune-based-therapies-to-its-treatment-profile-639654/ March 2015).

VG-1000 vaccine: This vaccine is most beneficial in treating carcinomas, leukaemia, and melanomas, and it is also suggested for some sarcomas (cancers of muscle, bone, and connective tissue). It is a medical product from natural placenta and can suppress tumour metastases, increase immunity, and accelerate tissue regeneration.

'Introduction of placenta extract results in destroying the protection system of the malignant neoplasm from immune response of the tumour host. If the organism and the immune system of oncological patient have not been damaged yet by beam-therapy and chemotherapy, the expressed response- the induced regression (disappearance) of the malignant tumor is observed' (http://www.limbt.com/page/35/, March 2015).

5. Psychology, Hypnosis, and Psychotherapy

Although these are used at most clinics, they are considered adjunctive therapies. 'Psychological counselling, support groups and even psychotherapy make up a critically important aspect of therapy in the world's most successful cancer treatment centres. Some doctors have reported that a traumatic psychological event in a person's life may trigger the appearance of cancer one to two years later. Music, meditation, relaxation techniques, and stress reduction have proven to significantly enhance the power of the immune system. Some therapists include emotional and even spiritual counselling, not only for the person's regular life, but in dealing with the trauma of cancer.'(http://www.cancure.org/choice-of-therapy;March 2015).

Those are some alternative cancer treatments, but not all of them, and as you see, there are many of them to choose from. You just need to find the one, or more, which you (and your doctor) like and feel comfortable using.

Don't forget that we are living in a fast-evolving world with a compound system of increase in consciousness and that in every year there will be new discoveries and treatments to help you in the fight against cancer. Stay connected with the science, books, and the Internet and you will be victorious.

Testimonies

I wish just to remind you a few books and articles (already presented here), which have empowered and helped me in my fight with cancer. There are beautiful stories about people which, like me, have been sent at home to die and they save themselves through faith and perseverance:

Anita Moorjani's *Dying to Be Me*

http://www.amazon.com/Dying-To-Be-Me-Journey/dp/1401937519

http://www.youtube.com/watch?v=rhcJNJbRJ6U

Dr Lorraine Day's *Cancer Doesn't Scare Me Anymore*

http://www.drday.com/

Jannete Murray Wakelin's *Raw Can Cure Cancer*

http://rawcancure.com/

Dr David Hawkins's *Healing and Recovery*

http://www.amazon.com/David-R.-Hawkins/e/B001H6MLOO

Brandon Bays's *The Journey*

Claude M. Bristol and Harold Sherman's *TNT: The Power within You*

Claude M. Bristol's *The Magic of Believing*

Louise Hay's *Heal Your Body*

Barbara Brennan's *Light Emerging* and *Hands of Light*

http://www.amazon.com/Hands-Light-Healing-Through-Energy/dp/0553345397

Michael Newton's *The Journey of Souls*

http://themindunleashed.org/2013/06/using-your-thoughts-to-better-you.html.

Now, if you wish and if you have time to read a story about a tumultuous life of continuously fighting for survival, you can read the next chapter, 'My Story'.

I have made it short, as this book is mainly about cancer treatment, not about me. I will present more specific details in the next book, "Who are you? The Journey to Yourself", and keep you informed about the outcome of my treatment after years. It takes a lot of courage to unveil your life in front of everybody, but I thought that reading my story will help you to understand the cause of cancer and will give you an example of tenacity, courage, and faith, empowering you to keep going.

In all our small or hard battles, we need support and encouragement as a source of energy, a little battery or plug where we can recharge and keep going. And we need this positive energy more in the battle with cancer because of the imprinted idea from the society that cancer equals death.

If we can see or read about the great number of survivors that had conquered cancer, we will understand that cancer is nothing less than a normal disease comparable to diabetes or stroke. Cancer is actually just a big disturbance in our metabolism plus a weakened immune system, that's all !

Statistics shows that at every six seconds in the world, somebody dies from diabetes-related causes; in 2013 diabetes caused 5.1 million deaths, and cancer caused a bit more than diabetes—8.2 million.

So we need to keep a positive attitude and not see cancer as a tragedy or a dead end, but as a normal disease which can be treated and beaten.

I remember the positive impact of all the books and DVDs which Dr Coralia gave me and how they were my life preserver in the middle of the ocean for me. I will be forever grateful for her help. God bless her! Without those testimonies, I wouldn't be able to continue my fight and survive.

It is comforting and inspiring to know that there are people who went through the hell of cancer and came out victorious. That will give you hope and impulse to not give up in your battle.

Just keep in mind that if I made it, you can make it too!

CHAPTER 5

MY STORY

My story starts in the small Romanian city of Turnu Severin on the shore of Danube in 1960.

I will not waste your time with a long story of my life, and of course, I can't fit fifty years of life in a few pages of a book. But I wish to present the factors which contributed to the emergence of my cancer, as I know that many of you had the same stress and problems that led to the disease.

The year 1960 was the year of my birth and of communism's official birth in Romania. Although in theory communism offers equal rights to everybody, in practice it was a cage for the mind and spirit. The dictator—the president Georghe Gheorghiu-Dej and, later, Nicolae Ceausescu—closed the borders and isolated us from the world. Nobody had a passport or the right to travel abroad. On TV, there were only Romanian programs and movies; abortion was illegal, and contraceptives were taken out from the market as the country needed 'workers' to build communism. Land and assets were taken from people, and if some people opposed, they were thrown in jail, fed only with bread and water, and beaten until they died.

The land was possessed by the government, and the farmers were forced to work in collectives (collective farm) and paid with products. Patrols of five to seven policemen walked on the streets, stopping people and checking IDs. If you couldn't prove that you have a job, you would be taken away and forced to dig canals or work in the mines with very little pay. You never should stay in groups to talk, and always you needed to talk loud enough for everybody to hear the subject. The whisperers were considered as plotting against the government and were punished with jail or unpaid work.

Through terror and punishment, they forced everybody to work. There were no benefits for the disabled or unemployed. Everybody had to work; it didn't matter what. Disabled people had special schools and hospices, where they manufactured things for the community. People without arms painted with their mouths or knitted with their legs, and for some reason, there were very few disabled people around. Mothers had no choice but to stay at home with the kids for no more than six months; after that, all babies went to the nursery, which was free, as well as the educational system. The health system was free also, but because the salaries were small, all doctors and specially the surgeons wanted under-the-table cash for them to treat you properly.

All the institutions, factories, land, and animals belonged to the government. There were no rest homes, and families took care of the elders until they died. Corruption was the queen in all fields, contributing to the devaluation of human quality and dumping the kindness and honesty in the mud of egoism, hatred, and lies. The natural riches of the country were exported, and the people became poorer and poorer.

At one stage, for a few years before the revolution, nobody could go into shops to buy meat, sugar, oil, or flour when they wanted. Your name was on a list, and you got a ration, like in the war, once per month: 1 kilogram of sugar, 1 kilogram of rice, 1 kilogram of flour, 1 litre of oil, 2 small round breads, and 1 kilogram of meat per person per month. If you finished it before that, you had nothing to eat. The queue at shops to get the ration was so long that sometimes the goods ran out before you reached the line. Old people (all others were working) took chairs and blankets and sat in the queue from 2 to 3 a.m., sometimes all night, to make sure they will get some food for the family. All names were on a list, and you could sign and take the goods for all your family members.

When we got the products, I separated them into four parts and made sure we used each part no quicker than one week. I counted the slices of bread and the salami to have enough for each day to make sandwiches for the kids for lunch at school. In everything that we did, there was tension, aggression, and stress.

This was the environment I lived in for half of my life—a big cage where I, a scared puppet, had no right, no say, and no dreams, just work and tears. All of us had to obey and don't even think about the situation as it was no way out of it.

If you dare to complain, you ended up in jail and believe me, that Romanian jails were an accurate copy of the Auschwitz prisons.

And in this big cage, another one was made by my parents.

They came from a peaceful and innocent life in a village, where human values were respected and appreciated. They moved to a big city, a mirror where the hideous mask of communism showed its multiple abnormalities. Here, they perceived everything as a threat because everything was so different from their previous home reality. Their way of thinking was reflected in their excessive care for me, the only child (my mother lost a few pregnancies). I was not allowed to go out with anybody—boys or girls—so that nothing bad would happen to me.

The only trip, or party, I was allowed to go to in twelve years of school was the trip at the end of high school. Also nobody was good enough to come in the house to play with me; some of my colleagues who were more free in thinking were labelled as light girls, and others who were more religious were considered a threat to my orthodox religion. I had a very good friend, Pentecostal, who visited me a few times, but when she started talking about the sins of drinking, hitting, and swearing, they stopped her from playing with me because that was their way of living.

One day on our way back from school, we were talking at the crossroads before saying goodbye, and my father drove pass and saw us. He said from the car's window, 'We'll talk when I come home.' That meant to be ready to be beaten. I was very scared, and I was praying to God to protect me; that was the first time when I had a vision of Jesus walking on water towards me and hugging me.

Indeed, when my father came home, I was beaten with the belt so bad until I lost consciousness just because I was talking with a Pentecostal girl when I was told to not to.

My father had a very hard life. He grew up with a stepmother, a very bad one, and a very aggressive father, who always beat him with the whip and the belt. As a child, he had no shoes, and his clothes were made from thick hemp; he looked after sheep from 4 a.m. till 7 p.m. daily, walking many kilometres to take them to the pasture and back, eating only a piece of bread all day.

To escape from this hard life with his family, he ran away from home at twelve years old and started working in a truck garage, washing trucks. From there, he learned to drive all types of cars and became a professional driver. His actions with me, were a reflection of his childhood, but in other ways, he had a golden heart, and he would give his life for me.

My mother lost her father on the war, before she was born. Her mother had a lot of land and workers to take care of, and my mother grew up mostly alone without much love or care. She never knew how to get close to me to share love or to be my friend. Her only worry was what people would say about us.

So based on their backgrounds, both my parents tried to protect me from some imaginary dangers. They put me in a second cage, a cage of isolation, loneliness, and sadness, burying in me any ability to connect and socialize. They even chose my husband. None of the boys who wanted to be my friends were good enough for them. I was in love with a very handsome guy, but because he had darker skin, they called him gipsy and stopped him from passing on our street. He waited for months in the rain and snow at the corner of the street, hoping to see me in the backyard. After a while, he gave up.

My mother chose for me one of my high school colleagues because he had a father who was a colonel in the army, a mother who was a nurse, and he was planning to become a doctor. She didn't care when I told her that he didn't like kids and animals and that he was a sadistic man. He has put his dog in chains and throw at him knives or paper cones with needles on top and has poured petrol on a cat's tail and set her on fire. She liked him, because he brought flowers when he visited and was well mannered, but most of all, she liked the idea that he would become a doctor and we would be rich.

After I finished high school, I searched for a university as far as possible from home, thinking that when I finish, I would disappear and escape from her dictatorship.

While I was making plans to escape, she at home was making plans for my wedding, telling all neighbours that when I finish university, I will get married.

To be honest, I liked him because he was a very handsome guy and we were neighbours and school colleagues for seven years. But I couldn't say that it was mad, blind love, and I don't think that he loved me at all, just wanted to have fun. We visited each other, and in one weekend, his parents came to my parents to discuss our relationship. My mother was happy that her dream would come true.

I was studying 2,000 kilometres away and still had two years to go, and in every holiday, we were together. Unfortunately for all of us, in one visit, I become pregnant, and because I kept my dream to be free and go away, an aunty helped me to make an abortion at his home. When my parents found out, they became completely hysterical, and of course, they started to beat me with the belt. Somehow, I escaped with my clothes torn, so sick and full of blood and I ran barefoot at night to him. They followed me there and started an argument with him and his parents, threatening us that my mother would give us all to the police because we made an illegal abortion and I may never be able to have kids because of that.

I felt then that all my life is a mistake, and I wanted to die to end everything. My mother, who should have been on my side to protect and comfort me in that crucial moment, was my executioner. My heart was broken to hundreds of pieces by the guilt of taking a life, the pain of being rejected and accused by my own mother, and the anger of a forced marriage. It was an entire show, and we ended up promising that we would marry as soon as possible. The next day, I had a terrible haemorrhage, and I almost lost my life because the doctors didn't want to operate on me unless I told them who performed the abortion so he or she could be put in jail.

I lost consciousness, and for a few days, I was in a coma, with transfusions and perfusions. Two weeks later, he took me home, and we started planning the wedding. The next day after the wedding, we left the city, as I had a position as biology teacher in the north of the country. For one year, my parents didn't know where I was, and I refused to talk with them. After they found us, they came and brought some clothes and asked us to end the animosity. Since then, our relation was cold and distant, especially between my husband and them. For me, they became some strangers who never cared about my feelings, and really, they never once asked me, 'How are you feeling?' or 'What you would like to do?' They decided, and I executed. They dictated to me to get married, and I executed, entering the third cage of my life: a cage of regrets, stress, and unhappiness.

For four years, I didn't get pregnant because I was thinking of divorce and also because my husband didn't like children. I took contraceptives continuously for ten years, different brands every time (it was very hard to buy them from the black market), as my husband didn't want to use any other protective method. My cancer was hormonal induced/dependent.

The village where I was a teacher was a jewellery of nature. The school was close to shops, the train, and mountains. We found accommodation in an amazing field sprinkled with flowers of all colours, at the edge of the mountain, between the forest and a creek. The owner came in every morning before I went to work and brought in the firewood and fresh milk from her cow. My husband didn't have a job.

The village, house, and school formed a little paradise, and it was the only joy I had in many years.

The feeling of freedom was overwhelming; I was finally free to earn my own money and be independent. My dream was joyful and real, and for a short time, I experienced real happiness. Unfortunately, I gave it away in caring more about others than me and obeying what others dictated to me.

At school, I decorated the classroom with didactic material, arranged a terrarium and an aquarium, making a great impression on my teacher colleagues. It was my first biology class, and I was proud that at twenty-four years old, I was able to spread the light of knowledge to others. Everything was ready, and a few days before the start of the school, I asked the school director if he had a relief teaching position for my husband. He was studying physics, anatomy, and chemistry to prepare for the exams for the school of medicine. He had tried to enter four times while I was at university, but he didn't pass the exams, and he thought that maybe if he was forced to write and explain the lessons to the kids, he would memorize them better for the exam.

The answer from the director was positive: yes, there was a position for a chemistry/physics relief teacher in a school a few kilometres away on top of the mountain, at 2,000 kilometres in altitude. The condition to offer him that position was for me to take the principal's position to that school lost in the wildness. The school was big and new; it had two levels, more than 300 students from year 1 to 10, and fifteen teachers. The problem was that no car could drive there, only 4WDs and the trucks, and in winter, not even those could climb the mountains, as the path was through the forest and on high rocks.

The village, named Lupcina (derived from *lup*, 'wolf'), was one of the few which communism couldn't collectivize due to the harsh life condition. Situated on the border with Ukraine, it was spread on hundreds of kilometres, and you needed to walk for hours to reach from one house to the other. People spoke a combination of Ukrainian and Romanian language, and their most important activity was drinking. Between their drunkenness, they shepherded the cattle.

To convince us to take the offer of living there, the local council offered us free accommodation, electricity and gas bottle for cooking, wood, and water, so we accepted.

We signed a three-year contract, and my husband promised that we would stay until I finished these three years of internship. After the three years of pedagogical practice, you could teach anywhere in the country, but not before that.

It broke my heart to leave my little paradise in the first village, but I thought that I should help him reach his dream too—to learn better and pass the exam at the school of medicine.

The principal's duty was not easy at all, and I couldn't ask too much from the kids and teachers in those conditions. They hardly spoke Romanian, and the primary school was taught in both languages: Ukrainian and Romanian. In winter, when the snow was over 1 metre, the school was closed. Most of the time, there was snow there because of the high altitude. The poor kids came to school by walking for one to two hours through snow over their knees. Their boots and pens were wet and frozen, and some of them were so poor that they didn't even had socks on their feet. Some of them were so tired after walking so long in the cold that they fell asleep when they reached the warm classroom.

In that winter, I lost a teacher, who was eaten by wolves; we found only the boots with the feet in them and the purse. Since then, I didn't cut the pay or penalize anybody by not reaching the school in time; I covered them in class, and I didn't report the absences to the head office. The teachers were very happy.

For a few months, our life was exciting there, discovering new places and people, learning new skills, and experiencing the country life. After the magic disappeared, my husband got bored or maybe homesick, and he stopped cutting firewood, stopped carrying water from a fountain ten minutes away. He stopped teaching in class, instead going on the sports field and playing soccer with the kids or going fishing.

We were fighting every day over almost everything. He replaced my name with Ms Principal. 'Ms Principal, serve the dinner', 'Ms Principal, wash my feet, make the fire', etc. He was aggressive, arrogant, and unhappy more and more. Before the end of the second year, one night, he said, 'I am going home. If you want to come with me, start packing the suitcase, as we are leaving tomorrow.'

You can imagine the arguments and discussions following that. I had sacrificed my paradise for him to help him to study, and now he was destroying my career by breaking the three-year contract. Without the compulsory three-year practice after the University, you would lose the right to teach, and there was no way to get a contract in the city, especially in our big city. I had to choose between marriage and career in that harsh condition. I was too scared to live with drunk and wild people by myself, so I decided to go back with him, with my heart bleeding.

In Timisoara, our home city, I found a job in a hospital for contagious diseases, Victor Babes Hospital, and I started studying medical laboratory for three years while I was working. My husband was changing jobs one after another, complaining at each one of them. When I brought the envelope with my salary payment at home, he took all the money, saying that he would do the shopping and pay the bills, but instead of that, he bought clothes for himself and electronics for music, which was his hobby.

My parents were paying our rent, and his parents were buying food for us; nobody could convince him to find a job and stop spending my salary. I was wearing second-hand clothes offered by my mother-in-law, and he had new clothes bought with my salary. Tension and arguments over everything continued, as we had such different ways of seeing life.

Every day, I was thinking of divorce, and when I brought in that discussion, he said, 'First, I will mutilate you with a knife [he had a

great addiction to knifes] to make sure nobody will marry you again.'
I even asked my parents to let me borrow money for the divorce, but
they refuse me, saying that in time he would change and his childish
behaviour would not last.

We were twenty-five years old, but he never changed.

After four years of marriage, I became pregnant by accident while I was
taking contraceptives. I had my period until the baby was four months,
and it was too late to have an abortion. Our first son, Adrian, was a
beautiful, healthy child, but my husband never touched him. I washed
all the nappies by hand (at that time, there were no disposable nappies),
cooked, cleaned, shopped, and took care of the kid and my husband
all by myself, while he listened to music with the headphones on. If I
argued with him and asked him to help me, I was beaten. When I went
back at work after six months, his parents and grandmother took care of
the kid. He didn't care and never changed a nappy or fed the kid even
when he was at home without working.

One time when the kid was sick and was crying more than usual, he
took him by one foot and hung up him out the window with the head
down (we were living on the fourth level), saying that if I couldn't
make him stop crying, he would throw him down. I fell on my knees
and begged him not to do it, and we argued for a few minutes. Our
neighbours watched that horrific scene from their windows, alarmed
by the kid's screaming. In that moment, I swore to myself that I would
never have another child with him and I would divorce him as soon as
possible.

Our relation become colder and colder, but I had no right to say no to
having sex, or I would be beaten. Two years later, I became pregnant
again despite the contraceptives, and I found out only at three months.
A young doctor from my work told me that she usually did abortions
by taking a whole pack of contraceptives at once. At that time, abortion
was still illegal, and the contraceptives were still on the black market.
I took the whole packet, and I almost died, but I didn't lose the child.

Our second child, Antim, was born with a malformation in the digestive tube and had a very hard life for two years; the doctors said that it was impossible to operate on him. My mother helped me to take care of him until he died at two years old. Antim's death changed my husband's behaviour and made him to feel guilty. He became the dad and husband which he should have been. I felt like a criminal, and I never forgave myself for that mistake. I prayed to God to forgive me, and I promised that I would bring another soul back—or maybe Antim's—and this time we would be the right parents. So it came to life one year later, our third son Theo, who was beautiful and healthy.

After Antim's death, things calmed down and went the right way. Having a function in the hospital's union, I found a job for my husband in the administration department, which he was happy with, as he would be driving most of the time and had a sort of freedom to do what he liked without being controlled.

Then started the revolution in our city to get rid of communism; we were living in Timisoara, the city where the revolution started. At that time, I was at home with the baby, and my husband was working. The hospital received tonnes of goods from Germany, France, Hungary, and other European cities for the staff and patients.

My colleagues sent a lot of goods for me via my husband and kept calling and asking if I liked them, but most of them I didn't receive. I thought that he may have taken them to my mother-in-law, but she didn't receive them either. Two of my colleagues were intrigued by this mystery and promised to find where he was taking the food and clothes instead of bringing them home to his kids.

It was the end of the summer, and my husband said that he wished to paint the apartment, so both kids and I went to stay with my parents at their holiday home in the mountains. After one month, I wanted to come back home because in the mountain, the winter starts earlier and it was too cold and raining for the kids there, but he said that he hadn't finished painting as he had gotten a second job and he was very busy.

When he didn't call me for my birthday, I thought that it was more than a job, so one day, without telling him, I asked my father to take me home, and I was surprised to see that he hadn't touched the paint on the apartment. His explanation was that he had a night job as a security officer for a shop newly opened and he wished to save that money in a separate account to take me on a holiday in Europe as now, after the revolution, the borders were open and, in ten years of marriage, we went only in one holiday to the Black Sea.

I believed him.

So his program started in the morning: had shower, left for work at the hospital, came home at 3–4 p.m., ate, showered, changed clothes, and left for the second job. I saw him the next day in the morning when he started the same ritual. And I believed him until one day those two colleagues from work came to see the kids and told me that he had a mistress and that every day after work he went there and that the other job didn't exist.

I felt that all the burden and sacrifices of ten years of marriage were wasted in vain, but at the same time, I felt that this was the moment when I should do something for my freedom. I went to a friend who was a lawyer and told her the situation, and she agreed to represent me without money and to pay her when I was free and had managed my money.

One day I changed the locker on the door and asked my parents to stay with me. When he came home to shower and go to her, I gave him the divorce papers and asked him to pack his clothes and go. He had fallen into a trap and didn't have a way out. Because his father had big connections in the corrupted field of the court magistrates, he tried to take my apartment, which I received from work and paid with my salary, to throw me and the kids out on the street, but my lawyer told me what to do. My father paid the remaining mortgage, and I kept the apartment. Then his father tried to take my older son, Adrian. My father-in-law had throat cancer and was saying that he wanted to adopt my son. He would die soon, and the child would have a survivorship pension from him. I told him that my kids were not for sale, as I knew that if he had this right, he would never let me see or be with my child. He started a plot to be able to take Adrian by law, but he died before reaching his plan.

Again, I had only God on my side on this fight. Since then, my husband never came to see the kids and *never* sent a dollar to them even when he was later living in America. I tried a few times to get child support in court, but they couldn't find him. Although his mother kept in touch with us, sending some presents for the kids' birthdays, she never told us where he was. I heard stories that he was giving tips of hundreds of dollars to the waiters at the restaurants, but he never thought to save or send a dollar to his kids and I never understood his inhuman behaviour. So I raised the kids alone without any financial help from him, his family, or the government, working most of the time two jobs—one full time at the hospital and a casual one at the local television station Europa Nova, doing marketing with my friend Christina M.

This was the end of the third cage in which I was living, but it took me three years to enjoy the freedom. To escape from the past, I decided that I needed to leave the country, my parents, and all those bad memories, to run far away from those three cages in which I was forced to live. The problem was that I didn't have any money, and the only way to emigrate was to marry a foreigner. I tried on the Internet, and I went to Pentecostals' and Jehovah's Witnesses' churches. I met a very handsome man with three kids, who was thinking to go to Germany also, but his ex-wife didn't give him the consent to take the kids away. We lived together for one year until I found that his son had some mental problems (he tried to kill his other three brothers and sister and himself a few times) but that his father refused to treat him. It was a year of stress and dramas, and I will describe them in the next book just for you to see how much the human body and mind can take before having a 'strike' called cancer.

I broke up with him, and in the same day, after coming back from the court, the head of the regional union where I was representing Victor Babes Hospital sent reporters from Holland to my home (because I could speak English) to get some information about the post-revolution development of the Romanian health system in the city where the revolution started.

They were a couple, Renee and James, very nice and professional, and both were reporters at the Netherlands. They took pictures with us and wrote down all the information about our salary and our problems in the health sector. After a few weeks, I received a letter with a page from the newspaper that had our pictures (the kids and I) and the story, word for word, that I told them. At the beginning, I was upset because I didn't consider myself a victim at that time, as I had my own apartment, a very good job, and a management function in the union. Then I thought that the interview was about the country, not about me, and later, I understood that in their standards, we represented the country and we were in a big mess, living under the Western European standards. They took me and my elder son, Adrian, for a visit to Holland, and we travelled and were hosted by a few different families who were impressed by our story. We met very kind and rich people, and it was an amazing experience. After that visit, Renee opened a bank account in Holland for me, and many people whom I'd never met sent us money and parcels for more than one year. That was God's hand sending us money to pay for the emigration.

I was afraid to tell my parents that I intended to emigrate; they would do everything that they could to stop us because they considered Romania the best country in the world, and we would be traitors if we would leave. Without telling them, I acquired passports for me and the kids and sent five applications to emigrate to Canada, America, Holland, Australia, and New Zealand, planning to go to the one that would answer first.

And the first to answer was New Zealand. Other two friends of mine, Alina and Luci, had already left for New Zealand with their families. I received a working visa for six months with the condition that I had to find a full-time job in my field—medical laboratory. I sold the apartment, and one week before the flight, I took all the furniture to my parents, told them the plan, and we left.

My mother almost collapsed and made tantrums, but it was too late to stop us.

It was the year 2002, and the kids were fifteen and ten years old. That was our first flight.

The immigration agency welcomed us at the airport and put us in a motel where I paid $80/day, which was equivalent to my salary for one entire month in Romania. Then they forgot about us. The next day, I took a map of Christchurch and a newspaper and started to search for accommodation. Because I had no idea which public transport to take to see the different apartments for rent, I walked with the kids almost everywhere in Christchurch. Finally, we found a two-bedroom apartment, and the immigration agent helped us to move in.

For the first two weeks, we slept on the floor in our sleeping bags and ate on newspapers on the floor, as the apartment was completely empty. There was no heater, and we were using the stove in the kitchen to heat the apartment. The walls were made from oil-painted stones, and the condensation ran on them, causing moulds on the carpet. It was cold and smelly, but the spring started to sprinkle flowers in Christchurch parks, and we were happy even in those conditions.

Then I remembered what Renee told me before I left: 'Go to a church. They are always helping poor people.' I went with the kids to the closest Anglican church, and there we met wonderful people who helped us with furniture and clothes.

I became very good friends with some of them, and Miss Dawn Tilly, a retired teacher, become my 'adoptive mum'. Watching how the money from the sale of my apartment was going down, I searched for jobs in the newspapers and Internet, but without success. It was a surprise for me to see that what the immigration agency told us that there were hundreds of jobs waiting for me, was a lie. When I approached them, worried that my visa would expire and that I would not be able to get a job to apply for residency, they took us and offered a job in a dairy farm in Rakaia, a small village near Christchurch.

I was the only woman there, and it was a terrible shock for me to work from a white laboratory coat and sterile environment to rubber boots in mud and manure, having a common kitchen and shower and toilet somewhere in the backyard far from the little sleeping cabin. Extremely stressed and disappointed, I called the immigration agent and asked him to take us back to Christchurch. Once again, we needed to buy furniture and pots and to start looking for a job. Finally, I found a job in the microbiology laboratory in a meat factory in Ashburton, a small country town.

We were happy and safe. The house which we rented was very big, clean, and beautiful. We even had a cat and a veggies garden. The kids went to the school very close to home, and I managed to buy a car and learn to drive on the left side of the road. The job was in three shifts, so at night, the kids remained alone in the house. God only knows what scars that left in their hearts, that loneliness at night.

In the factory, there was a terrible smell of decomposed meat, especially on Monday/Tuesday, coming perhaps from the crematorium. I needed to take samples from the factory tools, table, and the freshly killed and skinned cows (still trembling). Surrounding the rooms were canals full of running blood, and the smell of death, blood, and suffering was making me sick every day. After that experience, I was not able to eat meat for a few years. In front of the laboratory was a lavender bush, which helped me survive, and I told my boss to take care of that bush because if it withered, I would leave!

I lasted six months, and after we got the residency, we moved back to Christchurch and started again looking for a job. In meantime, I was doing volunteer work in a day-care centre for people with Alzheimer's. Sometimes with the boys, we volunteered for the Department of Conservation, making tacks and cleaning the parks and forests.

All this time, we were living off on the money from Romania, as we had no rights yet, and I kept sending more than 200 job applications. After a while, I found a three-shift job as a caregiver at Mary Potter Hospice for people with terminal illnesses.

One night, instead of having eight staff members on two wards, we were only four—two on each level of twenty rooms. That night, I had a back injury and recovered after two months of physiotherapy. Two of the other staff quit the next day, and after a few months, the hospital closed down.

I started again to search for a job with more and more urgency and stress as the money left was very small and we had three mouths to feed and two schools, rent, and bills to pay. The piles of CVs became higher and higher, and finally, I understood that it was a vicious circle.

To work in the health sector (my qualification) in New Zealand, you needed a medical board registration, but to get the registration, you needed to prove that you had more than eighteen months' work experience in that country. The problem was that nobody employed you without a medical registration, but to get medical registration, you needed to be employed; therefore, you were running in a circle.

When I realized that, I felt betrayed by the immigration system, which didn't tell me that I could never practice my job in New Zealand. It was time to have a discussion with the immigration agency and the government.

The immigration agency tried to calm me down, but they put more petrol on the fire, so I end up having an appointment at the Christchurch City Council, where I took all 200 job applications with the negative answers. I felt very stressed, upset, and betrayed, and I told them that I had used up all my money from home, I had no job, I had no money to pay the rent any more or to feed the kids, and I was in this mess because of the lies of the immigration agency, which I thought collaborated with the government. I told them that I would go to the Romanian embassy in Auckland to complain and I would tell my story to my reporter friend in the Netherlands and the whole Europe would know what was going on here.

I was hitting the wall!

My strike had a good result, and after a few different appointments with the council's representatives, I received a full-time job in a cytology laboratory with the condition that I study and sit an exam in cytology in New Zealand even when I had full qualification from my country. They even gave me a cheap council house with a big garden, where we planted vegetables.

After two years of study, I become a cytologist, and the council took that as their success in the immigration field. They invited me (on their expenses) to have a TV interview, a press conference in Wellington, and meetings with the immigration minister and other officials.

I suggested in the interview, that they change the law and asked those agencies to offer accommodation and a work contract to people they bring in and not to put the immigrant in such a high stress as I had been in. To my satisfaction, after a couple of months, fifteen other immigrants—all doctors, engineers, and teachers—went on strike at the embassy, having the same problem as me. So they changed the law, and from then on, all immigration agencies were forced by law to offer a work contract and accommodation to the immigrants.

Mission accomplished!

Unfortunately, after five years, the laboratory (MEDLAB) where I was working closed down, and I had the option to move to Auckland to work for the same company or to go somewhere else. It was another stressful situation to take the kids from their schools after they just settled in and made friends and for me to leave all the friends I'd made so far.

We decided to move to Australia. My elder son left first for Brisbane to see how the life there was, and I paid for him a course in animal care at TAFE. He dreamed of studying marine biology, but we didn't have money to pay for the course, he didn't have any financial help from his father or grandparents, and we didn't have any rights in Australia. He found accommodation, and after two months, we took a few things and moved to Australia with breaking hearts. My youngest son felt the changes the most, leaving behind a very good Asian friend.

At the beginning, we lived in a shared accommodation found by my elder son with other ten students, which was far away from his school and my work. I found a job at QML Pathology two weeks after arrival, and I was very happy. We moved into a nice apartment closer to the schools and work. Everything was perfect until the laboratory moved from West End to Murarrie, on the other side of the city. Coming from a small city and driving for more than two hours a day to reach home, it was too hard and stressful for me. Adrian also found a job in an aquarium shop in the same area as my work, and we decided to move there, as we were losing too much time on the road. We found a very spacious house with a garden and a beautiful terrace in Wynnum, a five-minute walk to the beach.

We were happy, but Theo, my younger son, couldn't take more changes and became a bit rebellious after he met a rebellious high school colleague, Jack, who had recently moved (disciplinary) to this school. Being new, both of them became friends and started a series of adventure to my despair, like ridding the bikes all night, walking for long distances to a remote island, climbing the school's roof, smoking and drinking, missing class, and other adventures like this. It was a very hard time for me, and I was under a lot of stress, as I couldn't find a solution to save him from that bad influence which could ruin his life. Both of them gave up high school one year before graduation, and it took me a lot of work to convince him later to continue his studies.

After three years, a Romanian family friend from Gold Coast asked me to help them to open a business in metalwork and to be the marketing manager. I saw that as an opportunity to make money to buy our own home and also to take Theo away from that rebellious friend of his. I received a transfer to a small lab of the same company, and we moved to Gold Coast. Eventually, the connection with his friend became weaker and weaker, and it ended when his friend ran away from home for a trip around Australia and never called or came to visit.

When separated from his friend, he studied law and justice administration at CLJA College, finishing it with the highest marks. We were in Gold Coast for two years, and Theo finished college while he was working part-time in an automotive mechanic shop, which was his passion. Adrian studied and worked in different fields—like tilling, construction, hospitality, aquarium, reptile care, landscaping, and web design—until he finally found his vocation as a sound engineer. He became a well-known DJ under the name Digital Synapsis.

We made friends and managed to buy our own home after my parents promised that they would sell the house in Romania and come to stay with us. I was their only child, and they were getting old and had nobody there to take care of them. We made the plan that with half the money (in euros) from their house, we would pay the mortgage and build a two-bedroom apartment for them and they would live off the other half plus their pension. This way, the mortgage would be very less, and we all would be together, enjoying our family life.

The house was beautiful, with a big corner block of land that encompassed their apartment and a veggie garden. It was at twenty minutes from the beach and fifteen minutes to the mountain, with a view to a picturesque park reserve and a big creek. Surrounding the house were twelve palm trees, three mango trees, two papayas, and a big jackfruit tree. I planted roses in the front yard, and Adrian made a waterfall in a pool with fish. We renovated the kitchen and the bathroom ourselves and put everything new in it. It was our little paradise; it had two big covered terraces, where we held parties and celebrations and made a lot of friends.

I was working full-time at the QML laboratory, and on weekends, I was doing marketing for the Rometal company. Everything was going well until the economy collapsed and we were forced to close the business. I found a second job on weekends as a cleaner at the hotel Azura, thanks to my friend Elena, to be able to pay the mortgage, and the money was just enough.

Then in an excess of patriotism and stuborrness, my mother decided that she would not emigrate to Australia because she didn't know the language and she had no friends (even when I told her that it was a big Romanian community(over 2000 people) there and we knew four Romanian families already). For me, that was the knockout punch, and I couldn't believe what she was doing. My father wanted dearly to come to be with us. He asked me to send a boy to bring him here to see how it was, and he would decide after that. I borrowed more money from the bank, acquired a visa for my father, and I sent Theo to bring him to Australia.

After three months of discussions, one week before they should leave, my mother deliberately drunk so much that she went in a coma and they had to take her to the hospital. She knew that if my father was coming to Australia, he would decide to move, and she didn't want that, so she did everything possible to stop that trip. Theo came back, as his ticket would expire, and my father, with broken heart, give up the trip to take care of my theatrical mother. The next day after Theo left, she told the doctor she would go home, and she was perfectly healthy since then.

I was very upset and didn't speak with my mother for a few months. Then when we started talking again, she kept asking us to go back home, saying that she was praying to God to do whatever He could to bring all of us back to stay with them. She didn't care that we had our life, friends, and jobs here. Her only problem was how to have a carer where she wanted—at home—and nobody else's life counted.

One year passed with weekly calls and arguments regarding the immigration, and my father asked me to send again a boy to bring him to Australia, swearing that this time he would come no matter what. Another debt of $5,000, another visa, and another break in the flow of life for Theo, but this time, they both had a plan—to stop Theo from coming back to Australia, by bribing him. They bought him a car and a motorbike and told him that they would put their home in his name if he stayed there until they died—and he accepted.

That was another punch under the belt for me, and I cried a river, knowing the miserable life they were living there in poverty and corruption and the sacrifice they had asked of my son. Theo lasted there for six months, time in which I hit the wall for the second time in my life.

From such a tension and from seven days of overtime work with no break or holiday for more than ten years, the tendon on my left shoulder snapped, and I couldn't screen at the microscope any more. When I told to my mother that I had an injury which endangered my career, she said, 'That's what you deserve for leaving your country! Now you found your paradise! Enjoy it! God has listened to my prayers to bring all of you home. I am so happy!'

I couldn't believe such an egoistic manifestation coming from a mother. Her words hurt and remained as scars forever in my heart. It is hard to hear this curse from a stranger, but to hear it from your mum, it is indescribably painful. She was happy for our pain and distress. I had nobody on my side in this fight, not even my mother!

Also I had the bad luck of getting a very old and mentally specialist booked by the work cover agency, who overdosed me on cortisone (without anaesthesia or ultrasound guidance), hoping to put me quickly back at work. Instead, he paralyzed my left arm for a few weeks by touching a nerve, and I was told that I would never be able to fully recover. The effect of the shock and the overdose with cortisone was a whole metabolism disturbance. I had a cortisol level in the blood that was ten times over the limit, and all the hormones connected with the suprarenal glands (which secrete cortisol too) were chaotic.

To correct them, my GP put me on oestrogen even when I was postmenopausal, and I was feeling sick, tired, and depressed. I was going to the toilet every fifteen to twenty minutes because of the stress or probably as my body tried to get rid of so many toxins, and the pain on my shoulder was getting worse day by day. I must tell you that during all this time, I was continuing to work and screen part-time with my right hand until I had the same injury on it too, but this was fixed with a single cortisone injection made properly by another doctor. I couldn't give up the work, as I had no other income to pay the mortgage or to support us. I was by myself with a burden much, much higher than my power. That was what communism taught me—to work even when disabled—and that was what I was doing!

Visits to tens of doctors, physiotherapists, and specialists followed, and their diagnosis was post-traumatic stress disorder and paid me work cover compensation. Then, like a cherry on top of the cake, the cytology laboratory in Gold Coast was closed down because of the economy collapse. I was at home with very little money, a huge mortgage, in terrible pain, with the prognosis that I would never be able to work in a laboratory again, and with my parents stealing my son and praying to God to make my life hell in order for me to return home. A wonderful life!

I don't know where I got the power to keep going, but I started training in child care, hoping to find an easier job. In the meantime, I kept applying for jobs in cytology, and finally, I found one in Brisbane at Healthscope. For eight months, I travelled 200 kilometres between Brisbane and Gold Coast, driving and screening full-time with one hand (my left hand was still painful and with restricted movements). We were thinking of moving to Brisbane and renting the house, but Adrian didn't want to leave. He said that the only place he would move to, was Melbourne because there were more job opportunities there and it was a more cosmopolitan city. I stayed with my friend Deepali for a few months in Brisbane, and I rented my room and Theo's room. But the house was in a mess, and the boys didn't pay the rent, so I moved back home.

I was drinking four to five 300-millilitre cups of coffee per day to last, leaving at 7 a.m. and coming back at 7 p.m. and then cooking, cleaning, and washing. The coffee aggravated the water elimination even more, and I was getting more sick and tired day by day, as all the minerals in my body were washed out. Finally, I collapsed and quit the job.

Instead of taking a break to recover, relax, and go on a holiday, I started looking for a childcare job in Melbourne. I didn't want to lose the house; if I couldn't offer my kids a whole family where they could feel loved and protected, at least I could offer them a place to call home, where they could feel safe when they needed to. The bank was pressuring me to pay the house, and I didn't have a choice. Very quickly, I found a job in a preschool in Melbourne. We,(Adrian and I) rented the house, fully furnished, to a young couple, and we packed our suitcases and drove to Melbourne. We rented a beautiful house with a big garden for our dog Roxy, behind the Monash swimming pool. I was working full-time, and Adrian was studying sound engineering. Unfortunately, my hands didn't help me in lifting babies to change nappies, and the tendon snapped again. This time, I gave up! I felt that I had lost the battle.

The tenants in Gold Coast started to not pay the rent on different motives, my salary was not enough to pay the rent in Melbourne and the mortgage in Gold Coast, and I had only one hand functioning. I asked all my friends and connections to help me, but all had excuses.

The bank took our house in Gold Coast and declared me bankrupt. My dream to offer a home to my kids and my parents was over.

My fight with life was too much for me; I was alone with a burden too big and with no moral or material support. I was tired of doing Sisyphus's work, tired and sick. My body had enough of malnourishment, overwork, and stress without a break in fifteen years, and it had found a way to stop me from this run after the wind, from this madness of getting and having, but not living.

It created *cancer*!

In November 2012, one year after moving to Melbourne, I was diagnosed with breast cancer stage 3. I was fifty-two years old, and the specialist gave me six months to live. For a few weeks, I thought that this was the end! I couldn't think or care for anything, living in a kind of agony and careless attitude. The specialist, a sad and nervous Asian lady, refused to take out only the lump, saying that it would spread out. Her advice was to have complete mastectomy plus the lymph nodes removed, or I would need to find another specialist. I accepted, as I was feeling very sick and tired, and in 15 December, I was operated and had a DIEP flap breast reconstruction. Everybody tried to convince me to have chemotherapy because the cancer had spread to my lymph nodes, but I refused. They gave me six months to live without chemotherapy.

My life was about to end! The future didn't exist any more, and looking back, I couldn't see anything other than my two beautiful kids, who would become now orphans, alone in a foreign and hostile world, with no home, no mother, no father, no grandparents, or other family to take care of them.

In that moment, I regretted every second of my life, every second which I allowed to pass me by, without living and enjoying it, every moment when I was working two jobs or studying and not being with my kids or enjoying myself. In the movie of my life, I didn't exist—no pleasure, no joy, no love, and no happiness, only work, sadness, and a continuous struggle to make money, survive, and please others.

It was the time to ask *why*. Why did I suffer so much? Was this a punishment from God, as my mother had said? What would happen after I die? Was there a way out of this?

At that point, I had a long and vivid discussion with God, asking Him why. What had I done wrong? What was my purpose in this life? What was He expecting from me?

And He answered.

Before leaving Brisbane, I studied the Bible with the Jehovah's Witness family of Richard and Reiko, trying to get some answers, but I couldn't accept the idea of how the Creator could be so impartial to choose only a small bunch of people (Jews), caring for them only and killing or punishing all other nations for not obeying him or ignoring whole continents such as Africa, China, and India. I saw God as a universal force, impartial and life giving, not taking, and not a selfish, egoistic old man who will burn you eternally for some guilt created by the human mind to keep us in obedience for a time frame of approximately eighty years.

My god is freedom, love, and peace, and He is the life itself and the way of experiencing and enjoying life.

My god is not a taker. He doesn't take lives or make people suffer for not worshiping Him. He is content, as He has everything— the entire universe, all the power, everything. He doesn't need penitence or humiliation from anybody. He is the Almighty and doesn't care if a small tribe in Africa doesn't read the Bible; He doesn't punish them with plagues for that. He loves all forms of life equally with a pure, unconditional love that does not request a payback or bribes with prayers or worship. He was a giver. He was giving life and joy. He creates life continuously and wishes us to enjoy it and to be part of it. He is enjoying and experiencing life through us and within us in its infinite forms of manifestation. God does not suffer from jealousy, envy, egoism (to request absolute worship), or anger. He is at peace, kind, and loving.

He is *all* that it is !

In Melbourne, I met a Greek man, Michael K., who called himself Spirit Truth, and he answered all my questions about the creation, afterlife, soul, spirit, and our power to create our reality. For a whole year, he introduced me to the books of Dr David Hawkins, Eckhart Tole, and Teal Swan and to muscle testing, intuitive reading, light energy healing, and everything about life and positive thinking. I was learning and 'drinking' information like a dry sponge, and one by one, all my questions were answered in long out-of-time discussions. He woke me up from a fifty-year nightmare, and I can't be thankful enough for his teachings.

I will share all the subjects discussed in my next book about my journey, as you may have the same questions like I had, and it is good to know there is only one truth and that it can be verified and understood.

He taught me to say affirmations, and I created one to fit my life, but I didn't say it until later, after another spiritual friend, Chris, convinced me of the power of them. At the moment, I am using two affirmations:

a) 'The infinite divine intelligence is guiding me in every moment and in every way, and I am taking the perfect decisions for my health and for my life. The perfect situations and the perfect people are coming in my life, and I am happy, I am healthy, I am fit. I have everything that I want, and I am grateful for everything that I have.'

b) 'I am an extension of the mind of Creator, experiencing Himself in this realm of perceived reality and manifesting love, health, and happiness'

Michael introduced me to a meditation group coordinated by a naturopath couple, Rene and Karin, extending my circle of friends. He was opening a door to a magnificent world, liberating my mind and soul from the fear of death and the unknown.

That was the moment when I started living. My cancer was the key to a new world, to a different reality and understanding. I was awake from a long nightmare, happy to be alive and blessed to understand that I was in this mess because of me, not because of my mother's prayers or because of a jealous and vengeful God.

The Creator is just creating all sorts of forms of life, which are living according to the universal rules and creating their own life based on their thinking and actions. They choose how they live—as a winner or as a victim.

I chose to be a *winner*.

On the day when I had the operation, I was praying to get another chance to make my life right, and I got it. After the operation, the nurses kept drugging me with morphine, and I complained to the doctor that I did not need any injections any more. Then they gave me pills, but I hid all the pills and gave it to the kids to throw them away because I didn't have any pain. Thanks to Dr David Hawkins's books, I was able to welcome and 'dissolve' the pain.

It is an interesting approach, and I highly recommend reading his books, especially *Healing and Recovery*. That was my first experiment to test the power of the mind in 'dissolving' the pain.

I was operated one week before Christmas. The reception area and the corridors were beautifully decorated with shiny Christmas decorations. I told to myself that they were doing this for me, as they were ready to celebrate my rebirth. Maybe Christ's birth is a reminder to us of another chance, another year to be reborn in a new spirit. Unfortunately, the society transformed Christmas into a race of shopping and money spending, forgetting the real meaning of the event.

Next day after the operation, while I was lying in bed, a very strange and miraculous event happened. I found myself out of my body, up in the left corner near the ceiling, very light, free, and happy, watching my body and the room and the nurses walking on the corridor doing their duties. I didn't feel any regret or sorrow, just a big release and peace. While I was watching through the window from my corner, I saw projected on a sunny blue sky a white operation table and about six to eight people/doctors in white clothes surrounding the table. From their fingers came out a bluish-white light like long strings, which formed a net around the table.

My body was on that table, and I knew that they were healing me. Their face had a light -milk-chocolate colour, and they were very concentrated on their work. I was thinking that I must have been very sick if I had so many 'doctors' around me, but I wasn't surprised to see my body in two different places at the same time. I think that the one on the table was my spiritual body. It looked like everything was normal, as I knew everything and I didn't have any questions. Curious to see better what they were doing, I floated a bit close to the table. In that moment, one of the doctors noticed me and opened his mouth in a welcoming smile. A strong beam of light came out of his mouth, and scared, I ran back into my body on the bed.

Instantly, I was watching the window, but nobody was there any more. I knew that it was not a dream, as I could see clearly the nurses outside and my body on the bed. I could hear them talking, and all the actions were happening at the same time in the same place. That was a unique experience, and I was afraid to tell it to anybody for fear that they might consider me crazy.

After a while, I told to my spiritual teacher and my kids, and all agreed that it was an out-of-body experience.

The next day, I started walking and eating, to the surprise of the doctors. And in four days, the wounds on my belly, breast, and armpit were healed, and all five drainage tubes were taken out of my body. Four days after the operation, they sent me home.

I felt an inexplicable joy to be alive and an immense gratitude for having a second chance. Every second was precious, and I was eager to live it to the fullest. If I had money, I would jump in an airplane and travel around the world (an old dream of mine), but I needed to be happy with what I had, and I had nothing material, only a big hope. Two weeks later, I was dancing and celebrating the New Year's Eve all night like it was my first day out. There was no operation, no pain, and no cancer—only joy!

Slowly, the tiredness and sickness disappeared, and I was healthier day by day.

Centrelink's payment was not so much, and I was not fully recovered, but they kept asking me to find a job through a disability employment agency although the cancer operation was not completely healed and my left hand had restricted movements and I was still going twenty to thirty times per day to the toilet (my doctor called it stress incontinence). It was pretty upsetting to see how they were forcing me to go to work, a lady fighting with cancer three months after having two operations (on the breast and belly for reconstruction) plus having a permanent arm injury and a diagnosis of post-traumatic stress disorder. I knew a few young Australians, one of whom was twenty and the other two around thirty years old, who despite being perfectly healthy were playing the stress-and-anxiety game, sitting at home for years on dole although they were lying!

I was fifty-three years old with a life-threatening disease and three other permanent injuries, but they sent me to work. Somebody suggested that I should sue them. Three months after the operation, sick of the employment agency's harassment, I found a job in after-school care as a coordinator at Camp Australia, which required a bit of lifting (boxes with toys) and physical work, but I liked it. This job reminded me of my 'first love'—teaching—and I was doing it with great pleasure. We had a lot of activities and fun with the kids, and sometimes I had one or two assistants to help supervise them.

A couple of times, my lower back and shoulder were so painful, the muscles got blocked, and I ended up in emergency, but overall, I was feeling well. Slowly, slowly I forgot that I should enjoy life and do things which I like (painting, dancing, travelling), and I slid back into my old habits of working and overworking.

I started looking for a full-time job.

As I said, you just wish, and the universe says, 'Your wish is my command.' You make the choices and create the outcome of your life.

I found a full-time job in research at NIIM (Institute of Integrative Medicine). Always I dreamed of treating people using plants and reconnecting humans with nature. My grandmother from my father's side was a healer in her village, and I learned a few things from her and also by studying Biology. The head of the institute was Professor Avni Sali, and my boss, an very energetic and intelligent German doctor, was Karin Ried, who had a PhD in Genetics. We were doing a trial on garlic. The trial was to prove the effect of aged garlic on people with high blood pressure. I was searching for clinics to participate in the trial, sending the invitation letters to the patients, taking their blood samples, and measuring their blood pressure for one year—for 100 patients. It was a demanding job, especially because not many doctors were willing to recommend their patients, but I liked it dearly, as I wasn't stuck for eight hours at the microscope. I was working with people, and I was surrounded by intelligent and kind colleagues. But mostly it was because I was reaching my dream of connecting people with Mother Nature. After eight months, in one day I was driving for five hours in peak-hour traffic in central Melbourne to contact thirteen clinics as we could run out of patients.

I felt a bad pain in the right hip (the leg used for the acceleration and break), and I couldn't walk properly, but I ignored the pain. In that time, the institute moved to a new, bigger building, and I was packing and carrying some boxes too. Also, the lift didn't work for a couple of months, and I was climbing two levels on the stairs, aggravating the leg situation. The X-rays showed that I had three torn tendons, and the pain was overwhelming. The NIIM osteopath, Dr Simon Armstrong, tried to heal me and relieve the pain with a great dedication, and I was doing intravenous vitamin C, but the pain didn't disappear. He suggested for me to have a CT scan, which I did.

The result shows that I had bone metastases.

All the joy of a rewarding job and a happy life was overshadowed by this unexpected news. I remember Dr Amir Nekoee gave me the paper with the CT scan result without being able to say a word, looking with a deep sadness into my eyes. I started reading, and all he said was 'Don't read it all, just don't read it all.' There were a long list of multiple metastases to the pelvis, femur, and spine. I started crying, and he hugged me. What can you say to people who just read their death penalty? Nothing! The words have no meaning any more.

I quit the job, as I couldn't walk without a frame, and I agreed to do radiotherapy.

Probably, I wouldn't have gotten bone metastases if during the breast operation, the doctors hadn't cut a window in one rib to be able to connect the blood vessels to irrigate the transplanted tissue. Maybe . . . maybe I was doing the same mistakes as before, and that was why the situation got worse.

A full-body scan showed multiple metastases in the temporal bone, sternum, ribs, pelvis, and spine. With the diagnosis of terminal illness, the Department of Human Services gave me a disability pension. It was the last warning from my body.

After the radiation, for three weeks, I really felt that I would die. I had no power to talk or think; I was like a vegetable. I couldn't hold my urine, and I needed Pampers. I couldn't move from one side to the other, I couldn't sit or stand up, and I couldn't walk without the frame and sometimes not even with them. I slept only on my back, waking up all stiff and numb. All the bones in my body were in terrible pain, and every movement aggravated it. I was vomiting, could hardly eat, and my brain had something like a fog over it, stopping me from thinking properly. My elder son quit his job to take care of me, and he was doing research to find natural treatments. He was making me fruit and vegetable juices every day and drove me for the treatment and to the doctors, but most of all, he encouraged me and gave me hope. He reminded me that my grandmother was a healer in her village and that she cured a lot of diseases using plants and that we should use plants to heal me; he always had a connection with Mother Nature.

I felt that I had a second chance and I spoiled it. What did I do wrong? I was keeping up old habits—no special diet, no rest, no love for myself, just work and stress and thinking first of others and neglecting myself. Millions of other people were working harder than me but didn't get cancer. So what was feeding it? Then I started to research, and I found that my diet was wrong, my thinking was wrong, and my soul was full of resentment, grief, and anger. I was unhappy, stressed, and although my body was telling me that it was exhausted, I didn't care and put it through more hard work and stress.

But how was I to live in a society driven by money without producing it? I needed to work as there was no other option. I asked the Department of Human Resources to give me an apartment with a cheap rent, and they told me that the waiting list is between ten to fifteen years. There were other people too lazy to work who had been thrown out on the street by the landlords, and they got cheap accommodation from the government. I had no chance for an easy life.

From this amalgam of stress, grief for my parents' actions, malnutrition, and overwork, I was creating a shield, a shield of cancer, to stop myself from this crazy run and also to stop myself from going back to Romania, the place where I had so much pain and suffering, and to protect myself from again going through all that torture in my soul.

My moral duty to take care of my old parents was in balance with my fear of living again the same experiences in the past. Romania and my family were my torture chambers, and my body refused to go back to them by creating a protective shield. It thought, *If I am sick, they will not force me to go back.* But they did! My mother, in her egoistic view of life, told me that there were better treatments in Romania and that she knew many ladies who had recovered from cancer and that I must at least go home to die and be buried in my homeland. It didn't matter how, but I must go home—alive or dead!

I was sorry for her, and I tried to forgive her for her selfishness, but I am not sure that I did. I was very sorry for my father, whose health started deteriorating after this news, knowing that he had no chance to see me again, and he was torn apart between the dream of being with us and the duty to stay with my mother.

My son Theo left Romania and returned home, and he even got a job offer as a protective officer at the police. He refused and started an automotive mechanic apprenticeship with Kmart, enjoying very much what he was doing, working six days per week for only $7 an hour.

Every day I watched from my bed people walking on the street, people running, or even old people walking with a stick. My heart was crying, as I was not able to do more than a few steps inside the house. I bought a mobile toilet and put it near the bed because I was not able to walk to the bathroom. My pelvic bones and hips were welded, and the same was the case in the right knee. I didn't pray to live longer; my only wish was to be able to walk again, even a few more steps on the street or in the park, or at least to be able to go to the toilet. We had a beautiful park close to home, where I went before with my dog Roxy; now I could walk there only in my dreams.

That was all that I dreamed of—to be able to walk again!

My GP, Dr Coralia, started teaching me how to use natural therapies and provided many DVDs and books, which had a great impact on my healing. Also Dr Paolo Moraes from the Melbourne Therapy Clinic offered me a treatment with Iscador, a mistletoe extract which I injected on myself in the belly three times a week. I met a Russian girl, Lilly, who had a lot of knowledge in natural therapies because her mother had ovarian cancer. She shared with me all her research in this field, and I searched the Internet also to find natural cures for cancer. All this time, I had only one wish—to be able to walk again.

After a few weeks of eating only vegetarian food and drinking herbal tea and juices, I started feeling better, and I was able to reach the bathroom, walking with the frame. After two months, I was able to walk to the park slowly, sitting on the walker's chair on the way there and back as I was very weak and didn't have too much energy. For some reason, I could hardly breathe. It was a big day, and I remember sitting in the middle of the park, crying from the bottom of my heart and being grateful that I had another chance to be there and see it again.

That gave me hope, and I was determined to do more research and to collect information about alternative therapies. Always I was connected with and trusted in the power of nature; that was why I was studying biology in my country of origin. And because nothing was happening by hazard, I had carried with me from Romania a few books about the healing power of the plants, and I was using them now. Also my son Adrian started buying other books in this field and started being a vegetarian too, despite being the ferocious carnivore which he had been. I couldn't figure out if he was doing that from his conviction or just to support me in my fight. I ordered herbs and supplements from the Internet, and Dr Coralia kept me informed at every chance about new natural treatments which she found out.

That was how I collected all the information for this book, and I thought that it will be useful for others too, to save their time and maybe their life. If I had known all these things two years ago when I had the operation, everything would have been so much easier.

My treatment was simple and consistent. Usually in the morning, I would drink a smoothie made from vegetables and fruits. At the beginning, I used only the juice, but later, I put in blender all the veggies and fruits, diluted them with water, and drank the smoothie during the day. In the morning, after drinking the smoothie, I took vitamin B17 (one tablet), curcumin (two capsules), zinc, selenium (five drops), a tamoxifen, a Swisse Women multivitamin, or an adrenal stress support pill (from NIIM pharmacy), iodine, magnesium, vitamin D3, gotu kola, and sometimes some colloidal minerals and MSM. In summer mornings, I usually drank lemon juice in a glass of water with half a spoon of baking soda or Percy's powder, and after a few minutes, I drank the blended veggies. Sometimes I made a puree from polenta (boiled in water) and mixed it with cottage cheese and flaxseed oil, and sometimes I added plain yogurt to it.

I couldn't give up the eggs, which had always been my favourite, but I reduced them as much as I could. I completely stopped drinking coffee, fizzy drinks, bottled juices, or eating canned or packed food.

During the day, I avoided sweets, milk (replaced it with soy, rice, or coconut milk), meat, cheese, and pasta. Theo brought me two small blenders, and I was drinking blended fruits and vegetables during the day instead of water or having lunch. Also I had a bottle of tea made from camomile, calendula, herb Robert, Pau d'Arco, St John's wort, St Mary's thistle, *Chelidonium*, and salvia, and sometimes I added aloe vera to it.

In Dandenong forest, I found turkey tail mushrooms. I ground it in a coffee machine and added it to the food. My kids brought it every time they came home from camping. For dinner, I ate vegetables and sometimes fish and, extremely rarely, some chicken.

At night, I took again one tablet of vitamin B17, two curcumin pills and a mixture of tinctures from propolis, manuca honey, astragalus, cannabis, cat's claw, and sometimes *Echinacea*.

Slowly, the pain and the stiffness disappeared, and when I had pain on my legs, pelvis, spine, or sternum, I used topical solution of DMSO (without chlorine). I used it mostly on the sternum and the ribs where the surgeon made the cut at the operation because there appeared a hard lump, which was painful sometimes. A very useful topical treatment for bone metastases pain, is the following combination: a tea spoon of Turmeric plus half teaspoon of black pepper, one tablespoon of coconut oil(boiled before on slow temperature, for 4 to 6 hours with cannabis buds), one teaspoon of flaxseeds oil and a leaf of Aloe Vera (grounded). Mix all together, apply on a cotton cloth and cover it with glad wrap. Keep it on the skin over the night, than wash and do it again for as long as you feel the pain.

Three times per week, I injected myself with Iscador, and every fortnight, for several months, I had an IV vitamin C at NIIM Clinic, thanks to the kindness of the clinic's manager, Steve Bounce, who treated me with consideration even when I was not working there any more; otherwise, I wouldn't have money for such an expensive treatment, as the pension was just enough for the food and the rent. When I'm able to work again, I will pay back my debt to him.

Slowly, slowly my health improved. I regained my vitality and the colour in my face. I can't describe the happiness I felt when, for the first time in five months, I could walk again without the trolley or the stick. My neighbour, Hanna, a Dutch lady who was eighty years old and very active and energetic, kept me motivated to walk in the park with our dogs.

People at work and friends who knew me were impressed with my recovery, asking what treatment I was doing. I told them that I would write a book about it, and so I have done it.

Of course, all this time, I had ups and downs, and I had days when I was ready to give up the fight, especially after the radiation when I was like a vegetable, nailed in bed, unable to go even to the toilet. If I had the option to end up my life, then I would have done it without regrets. Everything was too much; it was all too much to make injections at every second day and to suffer that painful reaction to the Iscador, too much to prepare juices all day long with the last flick of energy I had, and too much to eat tasteless food and watch other people eat what they like. Sometimes I wanted to be normal and stop taking tens of drugs, and sometimes I had the feeling that everything was in vain and that we would die when it was our time to die no matter how hard we try to save our life.

At one time, I suddenly had a pleurisy, and for three weeks, I was in pain, with restricted movements. The most helpful treatment, apart from the antibiotics, was a cataplasm with a mixture of aloe vera, tumeric, medicinal charcoal, flaxseed (ground), and olive oil. I applied the mixture on the painful area, covered it with a piece of cloth and with gladwrap, and left it overnight. It had an amazing healing effect.

Someone who had a great negative impact upon me was a Romanian lady, Vasilica, whom I met during an IV treatment. She had breast cancer HER2+ with bone metastases, but she refused two years ago to take out the lump. She was in a continuous fight with her husband and her brother for her treatment. They were strongly against the natural treatment and pushed her into the hospitals, believing that was the right thing to do. When she was at home, she treated herself with natural treatments, but most of the time, they sent her to palliative care. She was in and out of the hospital for a few months, and I tried to help her, but her family became more and more unfriendly, hiding the supplements and harassing even her naturopath.

It was painful and depressing watching her fight with the cancer inside and outside and being alone in this battle. Every visit to her took me a step backwards in my fight with cancer, seeing her as the real proof that in the end, cancer will win. I saw myself in her in the near future, like looking in a mirror, and my heart was filled with a terrible anger, despair, and fear. I avoided her as much as I could, but on the other hand, I was so sorry for her to see that she had nobody on her side and her emotional suffering was much higher than the physical one. After a few months, she passed away, released from all those emotional and physical suffering. For a while, I was in much distress as I felt that I lost a battle myself by not being able to help her somehow, but I recovered at the thought that I had met her too late, when the cancer had spread all over her body.

Apart from the diet and the supplements taken, I continued to discover my inner self by doing meditation, contemplation, hypnotherapy, and different connections with the universal power—God. I discovered an organisation called the Unity of Melbourne, which had a great pastor, Bill Livingston, and where people had the same idea about God as I did and I felt welcomed and included. There I enhanced my spiritual baggage.

In regard to the hypnotherapy, I must tell you quickly a fascinating story, which I will present in detail together with other stories from this field in the next book.

In Romania I had a nephew, who was a successful hypnotherapist, Vlad Oprin, and he proposed to have some hypnosis meetings on Skype to see the roots of my cancer. He had cured prostate cancer and degenerative disc disease before among many other diseases.

So we started the session, and he took me into the far past, along a long corridor with many doors, asking me to open the door with the flashing light above, which I did.

Immediately, inside I stepped into a Peruvian plateau landscape of rocky mountains similar to the American Grand Canyon. There, three kids—a girl and two boys—were playing with a slide, close to the canyon. The older boy, at fifteen to sixteen years old, was pushing a slide from the top of the hill with the other two kids, both a few years younger than him.

I recognized myself being the Inca boy driving the slide. When the older boy pushed us, instead of using the proper direction, he changed the lane to give me a challenge to test my driving abilities. Instead of sliding to the valley, the slide went to the sharp border of the canyon, and I didn't have time to recover it. Both of us (the girl and me) fell down from a very high distance, smashing our bodies by rocks, suffering terrible pain.

The pain was so intense that I started screaming and crying in real life. My nephew Vlad brought me back on to the long corridor and asked me to invite all the kids in the story around a campfire to have a discussion. Then I understood that for a long time I had carried within me the guilt that I killed my friend, the girl on the slide, by not driving properly. Just now I found that was not my fault but our friend's fault by changing the slide direction. We had a discussion and forgave each other as none of us had bad intentions; it was just an unfortunate game. It was all overwhelming.

When I woke up from the hypnosis, I remembered that I always had a terrible fear of heights and I never was able to get closer to a cliff, being very disturbed even when I saw deep canyons in the movies. Now I know why. Also I had always a great compassion for the Native American

Indians, and their tragic stories of decimation by the conquistadors left a deep scar in my heart. Now I know why; in my previous life, I was one of them.

The interesting part is that when I looked on the Internet in that area where the event happened, I found the exact same image of the plateau near the Colca Canyon. I am planning to visit that region one day.

After the meeting, I tried to stand up to go to the toilet, but the pain on my ribs was excruciating; I felt like all my bones in my body were smashed, and I couldn't breathe.

I felt like I really had that accident. After the first step, because of the intense pain, I lost my consciousness and fell on the floor. I woke up a few minutes later surrounded by my kids and two ambulance doctors, who were trying to sedate me to take me to the ambulance. The diagnosis of the consultation was fracture of the right ribs. At the hospital, after many doses of morphine and blood tests, because the radiography showed no fracture, they sent me home. I had the pain for a few weeks; after that, it started to fade away and heal like in a normal, real fracture.

It was a very interesting experience, and if I hadn't lived it myself, I wouldn't have believed it.

Now it's been six months since I had the radiotherapy and started the natural treatment. I can walk, dance, climb the stairs, go for long trips in the forest and hills, and I am feeling better day by day.

At this moment as I am writing my story, I am in a nice resort, Naviti, in Fiji and planning to go to Peru in a few months' time after I help the NIIM to test a new device called ISET (the only one in Australia) for counting the circulating tumoural cells as my second qualification is in cytology. I won't go back to work, but I have a moral duty to the manager of the institute, Steve, to pay back his kindness of helping me when I was in need. Otherwise, I will fulfil my dream of travelling, relaxing, and enjoying my life as I should have done before.

Always I'm thinking that if the money is taken out of the world, we will have a completely different life. People will be more kind and friendly with each other, and the greed, egoism, and craving will disappear. There will be no competition, no war, no hatred—just peace and love. How nice will it be if the government will allocate a piece of land to every family and let them grow their own vegetables and animals, their healing plants and herbs. There will be no factories or pollution, and the humans will live in harmony with nature. Yes, that would be nice.

My first holiday after fifteen years of work and stress was possible only because I received my superannuation, as the specialists gave me only a few months to live.

I had not loved myself enough that I put everybody and everything else in front of me, ignoring my need for relaxation and rest. If you have cancer, you have probably done the same, and it is time for you to change! Remember that number one ingredient for curing cancer is *happiness*! Get out of all the conflicts and stress you are in, and relax. Do what you like the most, and enjoy being alive.

Fiji is the most beautiful island you can imagine. Everything here is peaceful and friendly: the people, the land, the temperature, the water, the wind, everything! There is such a positive energy around, and the air is so clean that you feel healthy the moment you arrived. People here are old fashioned but fully connected with the nature, and with their hearts pure and clean, not contaminated by corruption, greed, and hatred (most of them). They live in perfect harmony with nature, and nature nurtures them as the great mother she is. They are living in harmony and peace out of time, with no worries and no ambitions, just being.

I would like to live in this oasis of peace, and I am dreaming of opening a healing retreat here in this little paradise where I can put my knowledge about plants and natural healing in the service of people from all over the world. If I can heal myself using plants, than I can help anybody with it.

Here I found an eighty-six-year-old lady named Melaia Ratu from Vadraya Village in Korolevu, which told me that she cured cancer in her village using a combination of seven plants. I intend to try them, and I will let you know the result in my next book.

In the meantime, I give you the Fijian name of those plants just in case you wish to go there and try them.

This is Tarusila's phone number: 679.9160250. She is a niece of Melaia, and she will help you find the plants and talk with her aunt who doesn't speak English.

From Nadi Airport, you can take for $7 the bus which goes to Suva and ask to be stopped at the Assembly of God Church in Korolevu, which is close to the Naviti Resort (Coral Coast). Melaia lives in the house in front of the church.

For finding the plants, you may also get help from Ani, a nice lady living in Korolevu (phone: 679.6505020) who knows most of those plants.

Also, to identify them, you can use a book called *Fijian Medicinal Plants* by R. C. Cambie and J. Ash.

The following are the seven plants:

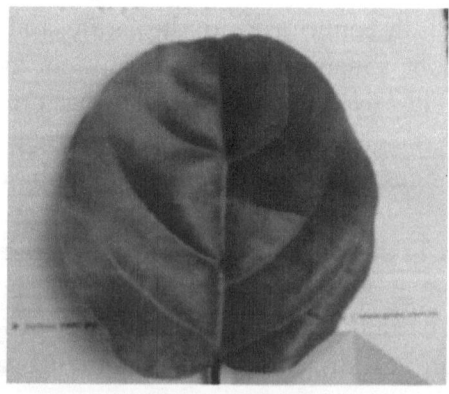

1. *Araro* or *kai hawa hawa.*

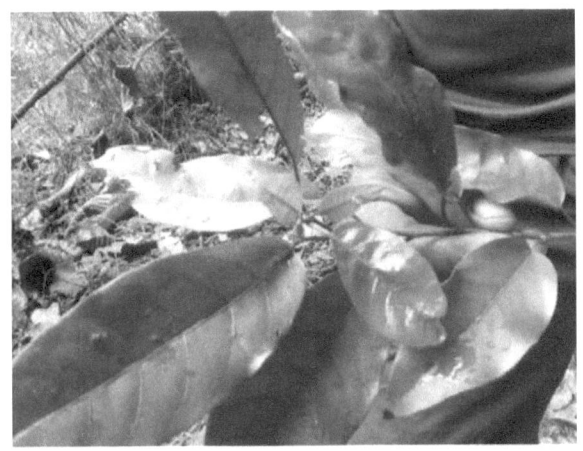

2. Cutumaruse.

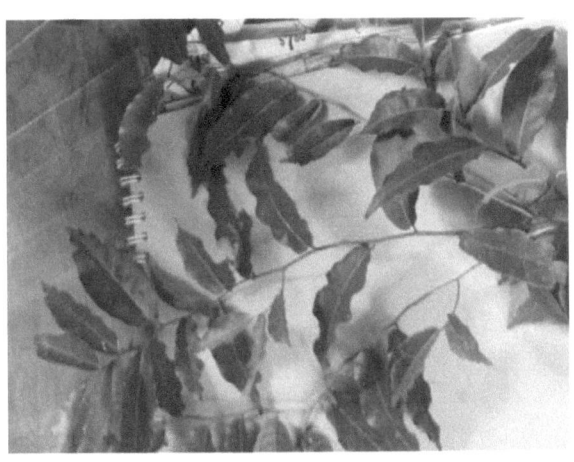

3. Masi masi.

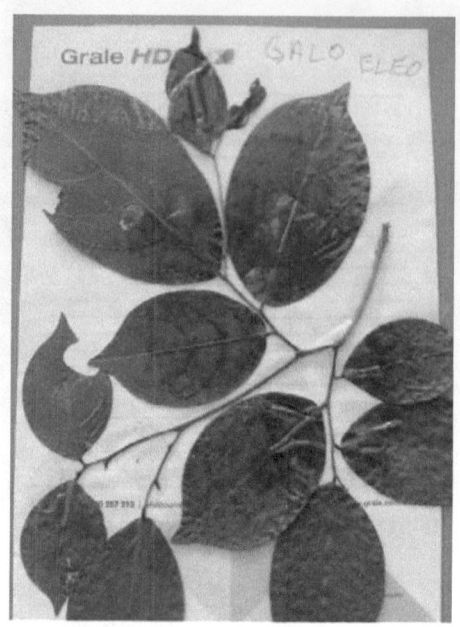

4. *Qualo eleo.*

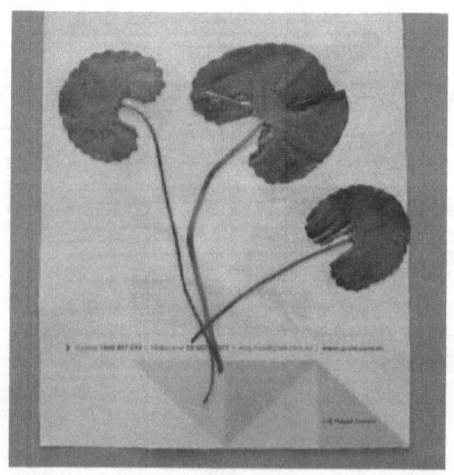

5. *Totondro* or gotu kola.

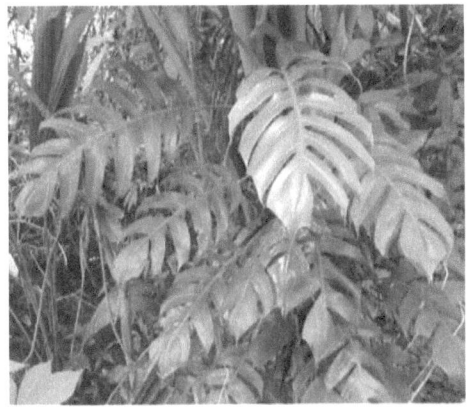

6. *Yalu.*

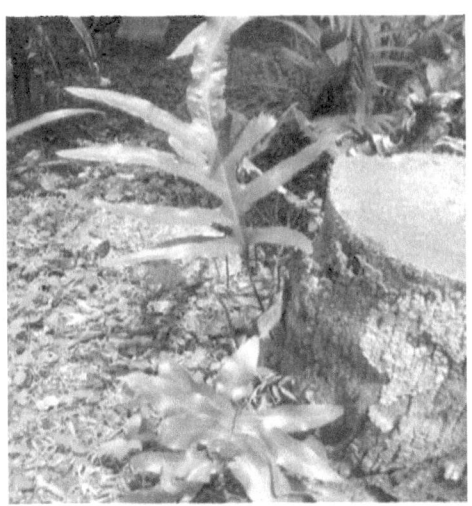

7. *Vati vati.*

If you can't find one of them, you can replace it with *kavika*'s leaves, which is a common tree in Fiji and has fruits similar to apples. See image:

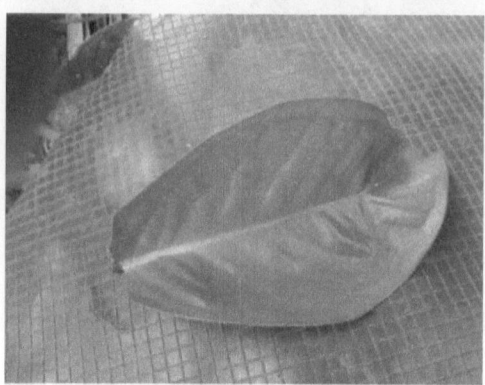

If you have any wounds on the breast or elsewhere, you can use topically a powerful juice from a plant called *tokatolu*. It is a liana growing on the beach sand with seeds like a small bean pod. See the image:

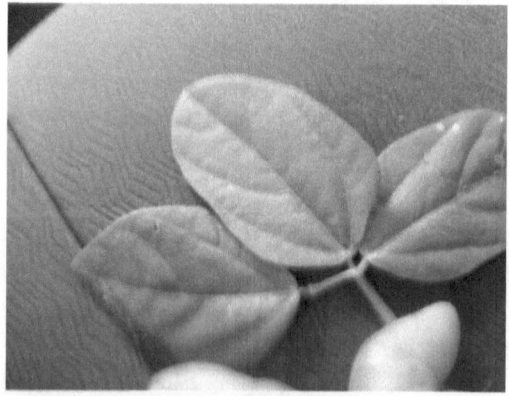

Also for the wounds, you can combine tokatolu and another well-known plant for wound healing: *wobosucu* (mile-a-minute).

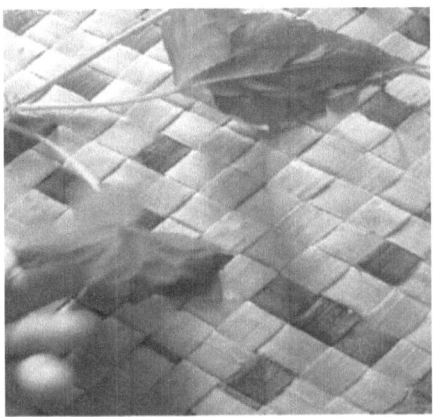

Each of the seven plants (only the leaves) needs to be blended separately (because the leaves are variable in size and you can't use the same number of them) with a small quantity of water and the same quantity of water for each of them. Take equal portions of the blended material and mix all seven together, strain it, and keep it in the fridge. You need to make enough quantity to last for four to five days drinking a cup three times per day thirty minutes before each meal. You can keep in the fridge the dry residue that remains after straining, and when you finish the potion, you can add more water to this residue, strain it again, and continue to drink it. That will be enough for another two days, making in total a treatment for one week. The taste of the potion is not bitter or sour. It has a strong chlorophyll taste, but not unpleasant; it is easy to drink.

Other sources say that the leaves of soursop/graviola tree (*Annona muricata*) the picture bellow are a very powerful cancer treatment. I also drank them blended with a bit of water.

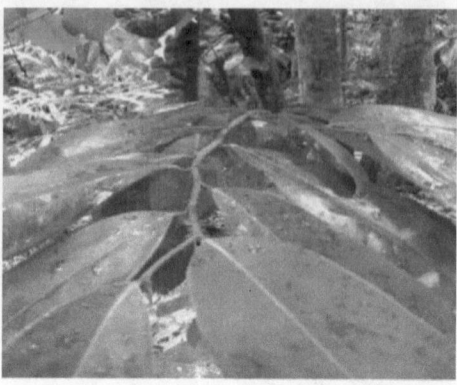

Melaia said that this single treatment (one week) will be enough to cure cancer, especially breast cancer.

Good luck!

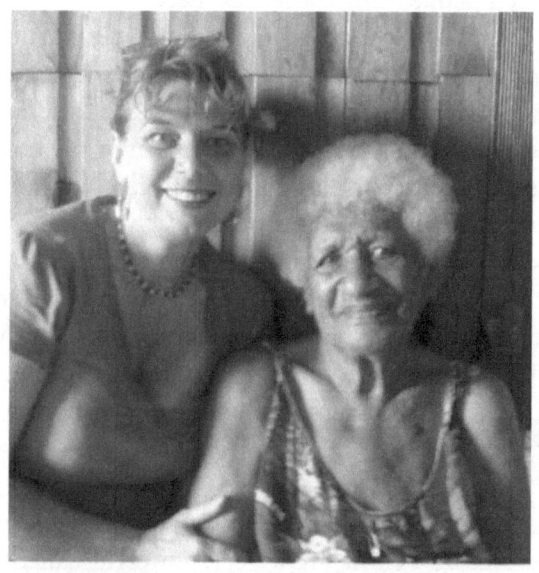

Melaia and me.

For any questions about the content in this book, you can contact me at angela45c@hotmail.com.

So this is a summary of my life story, and I have condensed the information as much as I could to not waste your time, as this book is about cancer treatment, not about me.

My reason for telling my story here is to show you that there is always hope in life and that even if you are knocked to the ground thousands of times, alone and without anybody on your side, there is still hope. Through all the struggles in my life, I had only God with me.

You have the whole power of the universe in yourself, the spirit of God, which can overpass any obstacles and all understanding. You just need to learn to use it, and it doesn't matter what your religious beliefs are. You all know deep inside you that there is a life force bigger than you that is keeping the entire universe in existence, including you, and if you will find a way to connect to that power, you are saved.

The only thing that you need is to believe and not fear cancer. Fear is the number one enemy in this world, and for some reason, it is propagated through media, advertising, TV, movies, news, etc. It surrounds us and keeps our spirit down. Your physical and mental health depends on your freedom from *fear*.

Jesus said, 'Your fait has cured you,' so *have faith, not fear* !

Claude Bristol and Harold Sherman said in their book *TNT: The Power within You*: 'Faith can move mountains, mountains of fear and doubt and worry, faith repeated again and again—faith in yourself, faith in the God Power within. It's a simple, silent, unspectacular operation, if you view it at any second, but over a long time span, what you accomplish will astound you.'

I hope that the information in this book will help you to take your destiny in your hands and heal yourself.

If things will go well and I will finalize my plan to live in Fiji, I will collect in a book all the information about the healing plants from the elders of the island, and I will offer you a tool to cure many other diseases and more options to cure cancer.

Until then, apply all the knowledge you have and find your inner peace and faith. God bless you!

REFERENCES

Moorjani, Anita, *Dying to Be Me.*

http://www.youtube.com/watch?v=rhcJNJbRJ6U.

Day, Lorraine, *Cancer Doesn't Scare Me Anymore.*

http://www.drday.com/.

Murray-Wakelin, Janette, *Raw Can Cure Cancer.*

http://rawcancure.com/.

Hawkins, David, *Healing and Recovery.*

http://www.amazon.com/David-R.-Hawkins/e/B001H6MLOO.

Brennan, Barbara, *Hands of Light.*

Fillmore, Charles, *Dynamics for Living.*

Bristol, Claude M., and Harold Sherman, *TNT: The Power within You.*

Newton, Michael Newton, *Journey of the Souls.*

http://themindunleashed.org/2013/06/using-your-thoughts-to-better-your.html.

http://www.myvmc.com/anatomy/blood-function-and-composition/#C3.

http://www.scribd.com/doc/205106778/Daca-Ai-Inteles-Acest-Articol-Ti-Ai-Salvat-Singur-Viata.

http://anthro.palomar.edu/blood/blood_components.htm.

http://www.innerbody.com/image/lympov.html.

https://van.physics.illinois.edu/qa/listing.php?id=17726.

http://sciencenetlinks.com/student-teacher-sheets/cells-your-body/.

http://quizlet.com/410483/cell-organelles-and-their-functions-flash-cards/.

http://quizlet.com/3064799/12-systems-of-the-body-whats-their-function-flash-cards/.

http://www.biologyjunction.com/cell_functions.htm.

http://www.naturalnews.com/021903_sunscreen_skin_cancer.html#.

http://www.naturalnews.com/021903_sunscreen_skin_cancer.html##ixzz3A5LOsaiX.

http://www.lef.org/magazine/mag2007/mar2007_nu_catsclaw_01.htm.

http://www.richardaluck.com/videos/creative-visualization-for-beginners/.

http://www.thedoctorweighsin.com/what-causes-inflammation-a-comprehensive-look-at-the-causes-and-effects-of-inflammation-part-2/.

http://www.msm-wholesale.com/shop_dmso.html.

www.cureyourowncancer.org/scientific-studies
http://www.greenmedinfo.com/substance/curcumin.

http://themindunleashed.org/2014/03/can-reprogram-dna-heal-frequency-vibration-energy.html.

http://youtu.be/75FQKQOKvVM.

http://www.mistletoeforcancer.org.uk/therapy/mistletoetherapy.html.

http://www.rense.com/1.mpicons/acidalka.htm.

http://www.oilsandplants.com/liver.htm.

http://realivzehealth.com/2013/09/24/lessons-from-the-mat-thymus-tapping/.

http://themindunleashed.org/2014/04/neuroscientist-explains-meditation-changes-brain.html.

http://www.ncbi.nlm.nih.gov/pubmed/22286244.

http://www.cancer.gov/cancertopics/pdq/supportivecare/fatigue/Patient/page1/AllPages.

http://beatcancerwithb17.blogspot.com.au/p/how-i-beat-cancer-with-b17.html.

http://viataverdeviu.ro/studiuinjectiile-cu-doze-mari-de-vitamina-c-anihileaza-cancerul/.

http: //drhoffman.com/article/intravenous-vitamin-c-for-cancer.

http://www.drlwilson.com/articles/COFFEE%20ENEMA.HTM.

http://www.ncbi.nlm.nih.gov/pmc/articles/PMC3655417/.

http://www.globalhealingcenter.com/natural-health/liver-cleanse-foods/

http://www.cancure.org/iscador_mistletoe.htm.

http://alternativecancertreatmentgerson.com/iscador-therapy/.

http://www.projectglobalawakening.com/2014/03/29/nature-of-mind/.

http://www.youtube.com/watch?v=rhcJNJbRJ6U.

http://viataverdeviu.ro/9-perechi-de-alimente-care-se-combina-bine-in-lupta-impotriva-bolilor/.

http://www.cureyourowncancer.org/how-cannabis-oil works.html#sthash.rGn8J0F9.dpuf.

http://www.innerbody.com/image_digeov/card10-new2.html.

http://training.seer.cancer.gov/disease/categories/classification.html.

http://www.health.harvard.edu/flu-resource-center/how-to-boost-your-immune-system.htm

http://pubs.acs.org/doi/abs/10.1021/bk-1994-0546.ch015

http://www.ncbi.nlm.nih.gov/pubmed/19276390

http://drsircus.com/medicine/sodium-bicarbonate-baking-soda/cancer-studies-ph-medicine

http://digitaljournal.com/article/323645

http://www.jcancer.org/v04p0703.htm

http://news.harvard.edu/gazette/story/2011/01/eight-weeks-to-a-better-brain/

http://www.massgeneral.org/about/pressrelease.aspx?id=1329

www.meditationonline.com/meditation

R. C. Henry, 'The Mental Universe', *Nature*, 436: 29, 2005

INDEX

www.ingramcontent.com/pod-product-compliance
Lightning Source LLC
Chambersburg PA
CBHW020736180526
45163CB00001B/257